HUMAN HORIZONS SERIES

LIVING
AFTER A STROKE

Diana Law and Barbara Paterson

C HD

love

Drana (Law)

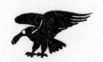

A CONDOR BOOK
SOUVENIR PRESS (E & A) LTD

ISBN 0 285 649140 Casebound
ISBN 0 285 649159 Paperback

Printed in Great Britain by
Bristol Typesetting Co. Ltd,
Barton Manor, St. Philips, Bristol

To God; and my dear family and relations, especially my 90-year mother, who dedicated her life to giving me strength and love; also my sister and her late husband, who were tireless in their efforts; to friends and scribes and the speech therapy profession, particularly to Joan Ellams; and to All Souls Church.

FORTES CREANTUR FORTIBUS

Acknowledgments

This book could not have been written without the help freely and generously given by Diana's family, friends, speech therapists and medical advisers. To all of them, thank you; and especially to the following:—

Jane Bedingfield
Reg Black
Bill Broderick
Jean Chiverton
Tony Chiverton
Doreen Cotter
Pam Court
Joan Crosley
Peggy Dalton
Rosamond Day
Barbara Deason
Betty Denny
Rosemary Duncan
Cyril Easterbrook
Yvonne Edels
Joan Ellams
Nancy Esterson
Isabel Freedman
Una Gavin
Betty Giles
Heather Griffin
Anne Handley-Derry
Marea Hartman
Bill Hepplewhite
Gill Hodgson
Michael Jackson
Wenona Keane

Gwynedd Laurie
Mary Law
Jean Lewis
Kay McDonald
Judith McLain
Jacqueline Morrell
Marianne Norris-Elye
Constance Offord
One of the
house governors
at Osborne House
Evelyn Penketh
Faith Porter
Morriss Rumer
Dr JDHS
Dr JGS
Daphne Stafford
John Scott
Dr A-M T
Catherine Taylor
Ted Taylor
Moira Tighe
Janet Wells
Joan Whycherley
Clifford Woodcock
Evelyn Woolf

It was not possible, owing to pressure on space, to approach all those who have helped in Diana's recovery; but to every single individual Diana wishes to express her heartfelt gratitude.

Contents

Foreword

Like most speech therapists, I had heard a good deal about Diana Law but, until I took office as Chairman, I had not met her. Our first contact was by telephone – the conversation was short, her vocabulary was limited but the message was clear and she made sure that it was understood.

In this book there are a number of messages – 'one of hope, laughter not tears' (p120), the value of a close-knit family, the rewards of determination, the need of a programme of rehabilitation – but perhaps the clearest message is to show the value of, and the need for, speech therapy. The frustration of not being able to say exactly what you want is difficult to cope with. Every bit of help is needed and it is needed quickly – delay just adds to the frustration and so slows progress.

Problems of communication usually do not arouse any emotion on the part of the listener except irritation. I hope this book will arouse sympathy and understanding for those who, like Diana, have a problem with communication.

Diana feels that she has benefited from speech therapy and the help she has had from speech therapists. The reverse is also true – we have gained. She has encouraged us by her endeavours; she has given us her backing and galvanised us into action on various occasions. Her pioneer work for the inter-denominational service has enabled others who are speech-handicapped to feel they are not alone.

I hope that those who read this book will gain an understanding of the problems faced by those who are not able to speak easily; and also by their families, who become so involved in the patient's rehabilitation.

Joyce L.Cook MCST
Chairman, College of Speech Therapists 1979–80

Prologue 1   'Life ... tragedies: but beautiful things between'

The small bed-sitter Diana Law uses in her mother's flat is a cross between an office and some kind of temporary army lodging. It's austere, almost impersonal; the non-essential ruthlessly pushed aside to make space for total dedication to her cause: increased help, in every way, for the speech-handicapped.

High up on the sixth floor, her window looks out only on to a brick parapet. There's a brass-handled chest of drawers, a small folding table, two chairs (one upright, one folding), a tall grey filing cabinet packed with tapes, letters, cuttings from newspapers and magazines. Her narrow, headless bed almost disappears under a heap of current work. A tangle of paper clips lies ready in a dish. The telephone, her much-prized essential link with the world outside, rings frequently.

On the table by her bed are bottles and boxes of pills, and a handsome lamp converted from a blue red and gold Chinese jar: 'bought from a jumble sale, my dear!' A small shelf holds a matched set of factual books on Ships, Trees, Birds – all prizes won over the years in competitive games at Osborne. There is no television either here or in the rest of the flat. Though sometimes she regrets it – she would love to be able to watch sport – she says: 'I have no time. Work work work!'

In a place of honour hangs a photo of Diana on the day

she received her MBE; next to it is her citation, signed by the Queen and the Duke of Edinburgh.

Diana moves around at surprising speed, with something of the rolling gait of a sailor. Her right leg is supported by the calliper made for her at the Wolfson Medical Rehabilitation Centre. Her left leg is slim and youthful, as her left hand is shapely and elegant, with polished nails and a seal ring; poised to dart into her filing cabinet, pluck out the right file, twitch out the right papers, flick through to the right sheet. Sometimes she takes hold of her other hand with a swift movement, and places it firmly on the chair arm or her lap, as though impatient with its unwillingness to co-operate more fully.

Her thin face is aware and mobile under the short shiny easy-to-look-after dark brown hair. Her expression is constantly changing, striving to expand her inadequate speech. There's never any doubt that a very active brain and forceful character are behind the alert dark eyes.

She talks slowly but distinctly. Sometimes a phrase comes tumbling out. Sometimes she takes a mental breath as she sees an awkward word coming up: 'Re-ha-bi-li-ta-tion': and she delivers it syllable by punctilious syllable. Sometimes she fails to capture the exact word she wants, and produces what she knows is an approximation with a matter-of-fact gesture. Numbers fox her; she goes through them in sequence until she arrives at the right one, or grabs a piece of paper and sketches it out with her left hand. Occasionally she gives up the search for a word, shrugs, gives a shout of laughter, and says explosively: 'My dear!' The slowness must frustrate but does not exhaust her. She has immense reserves of energy.

She organises her life and her campaign for the speechless with a concentration and single-mindedness many people both younger and fitter than herself could not begin to match. Files of letters to MPs, specialists, charities, wait in organised readiness. Copies of Hansard with answers to Questions on the disabled can be identified in an instant. Newsletters and leaflets about the latest ecumenical Service for those with speech difficulties, which she inaugurated, lie ready for distribution. Pre-addressed envelopes lie in a pile on the window-sill before being dispatched to local radio stations throughout the country.

It is difficult to believe that twelve years ago this lively, energetic woman was lying half-paralysed and totally speechless in a hospital bed; declared to be 'virtually an idiot. A hopeless case.'

Over Diana's bed hangs a picture painted by her mother in earlier days, showing a white bird flying above a wood of dark trees. Diana's temperament would never have permitted her to place it there as a deliberate comment on her situation: but, as her story shows, the symbolism is apt.

Prologue 2   Diary: Week starting December 10 1967

10	Sunday	Lunch 31	2nd in Advent
11	Monday	Sally G-S starts?	
		Reading	
12	Tuesday	Varsity Match	
		H 12.30	
13	Wednesday	13/pre Open Day	
		Lunch B. Water	
		SMA meeting	
14	Thursday	Xmas party	
15	Friday	Preston	
		Noisy fetch me 4.30–4.45	
		?night Harford	
16	Saturday	Ireland v New Zealand	
		Tube Invest.	
		?NZ v Barbarians	

Diana Law never went to the Christmas party, was never fetched by her friend Noisy, never attended the Ireland/New Zealand match.

At mid-day on Wednesday December 13th she was to experience the agonising headache which was the first sign of her massive stroke.

1 Early years

Diana Law was born in Sandycove, County Dublin, in 1919, of a staunchly Protestant family. Her father, a solicitor, died suddenly when she was only a child, leaving his widow with five children to support and educate. For her mother, Mary Law*, these were difficult and worrying years, but Diana remembers her childhood as a very happy time. She was sent to Princess Helena College in Hitchin, where she played an active part in school sports and eventually became Head Girl.

There were the two boys, then me, then Peter, then Jacqueline – a great surprise – five years after. We go bicycle rides in the country, long rides. Bathing, in the sea. Lovely!

My school a lovely school, but me, I was lazy, always lazy. I hated work. Every Sunday we learn the catechism for one hour, but afterwards I always forget! But I was always in the teams.

Always very active. I like tennis, golf, gardening, fishing, rowing, sailing. . . .

1939: FANY

Then came the war.

I chose the army because I like it. Not in peace, no. But in war, yes.

* see page 29

Diana joined up in FANY and went to Camberley for training, where she met two young women who were to become close friends: Daphne Stafford and Faith Porter.

Daphne Stafford, after her initial training period, was sent to the Middle East. After the war she took various secretarial jobs before joining the Foreign Office: later, as a 'very mature student', she took a history degree at Southampton.

Daphne Stafford. 'FANY is the Women's Transport Service; it was originally an early twentieth-century voluntary unit, the First Aid Nursing Yeomanry Corps. When the ATS was formed in 1938, FANY was partly co-opted into it to form the Motor Transport Company. It was paid by the Army, but did its own recruiting and came to be looked on as an officer-producing unit: not particularly tactful.

'Anyway, we both of us had great fun, though we were worked very hard. We were both clerks, really: Faith Porter was in charge of us.

'I didn't see any signs then of any great ambition! It was more of a good giggle at the time.'

Faith Porter served with FANY/ATS during the war. After demobilisation (the same day as Diana), she had various secretarial jobs in London; then took other jobs in the City before becoming, in 1962, secretary to the Headmaster of Eton.

Faith Porter. 'Diana made a great impression on us all when we first met up at Camberley. I can see her now. She turned up with bright red nails, a coat with a fur collar, and a very pretty silky print dress. She looked as though she was all set to lunch at the Ritz. They couldn't find a uniform to fit her, and she absolutely *refused* to wear an ill-fitting uniform, so for the next week there she was going round in her dress and coat while we were all being good little girls in khaki.

'She was a terrible rebel – she must have been just like that all through school. I shared a room with her for quite some while, and we had tremendous fun. She was the most original and dynamic person I've had among my friends. And she still is.

'I can remember. . . . We used to tease her terribly. When we were out there parading – for the Princess Royal I think – we were all there lining up, and in those days she had lots in front and we told her she spoiled the line, and then she'd sort of try to straighten up and we told her she stuck out behind. . . . She was a marvellous character.

'Very forceful. A leader. *Extremely* impatient. She never suffered fools gladly. Inexhaustible, and frightfully efficient. She did terribly well in the army. She was one of the first staff officers. Damned good. I've never known anyone with so much energy.

'She really burned the candles. A very full social life. Everyone had to jump to it – we all liked it. She was very popular. Never uncertain about anything. Dithering people drove her up the wall.

'She was aways a very active person. I never remember her sitting. She loved racing, and she'd spend days at Lord's. Her life was chock full. She never took up a needle, didn't knit, and you'd never see her with a book. Never dull, always good company. A black and white person.'

SHAEF: FRANCE AND GERMANY

After being commissioned Diana went on to work for SHAEF, first in Paris and Rheims and then in Frankfurt and Berlin. In Paris she met for the first time another life-long friend, Anne Handley-Derry.

Anne Handley-Derry, born in the Argentine, educated in England, took various secretarial jobs before joining MI(R) Branch of the War Office in November 1939. She was sent out to Cairo in May 1940 by the War Office, and after working for four years in GHQ Middle East returned to England in 1944. Later that year she became a FANY and joined SHAEF, first in London and then in Versailles and Frankfurt. In 1945 she went to Berlin as Personal Assistant to the Deputy Military Governor, General Sir Brian Robertson, and was there until the end of 1947. She remarried in 1948 and spent the next three years in France and Germany, returning in 1951. She has lived in London from 1956 and been in close touch with Diana ever since. She was awarded the MBE in 1947.

Anne Handley-Derry. 'I first met Diana in 1945 in Versailles, when we were both working for SHAEF. Later we shared a flat together with another friend in Frankfurt, from February to July 1945, and then again in Berlin, in the Grunewald.

'It was a strange time. Diana worked very hard – we all did – but she was an enormous party girl. Full of jokes. A great deal of Irish humour. Loved races, sport. . . . Used to chat away to the soldier who was supposed to be guarding us. Immense energy, immense drive. She could always cope with everything.'

However hard she played, Diana worked with equal ferocity. She was one of the very few women to attain the rank of Senior Commander (the equivalent of Major): the letter appointing her expresses the Army Council's 'thanks for the valuable services which you have rendered in the service of your country at a time of grave national emergency.'

Her scrapbook contains evocative mementos of these years: a pass to SHAEF Supreme Headquarters; a photo of herself in uniform, looking like a 1940s war film heroine;

a form letter from Montgomery on non-fraternisation; a 1945 Easter greetings card from the Mess Section of the Supreme Headquarters in France. General Eisenhower gave her a copy of the historic document announcing the end of the war, which he signed specially for her when she and his secretary, Kay Summersby, were both in his office a few days later. She also has the outgoing message from SHAEF Forward to AGWAR for Combined Chiefs of Staff and the AMSSO for British Chiefs of Staff, announcing simply: 'The Mission of this Allied Force was fulfilled 0241, local time, May 7th 1945.'

She was demobilised with the highest recommendations. Brigadier F. Field stated that, in Paris, Rheims and Frankfurt, 'she displayed the same characteristics of great energy combined with unfailing good humour;' while Captain G. E. Hughes (RN), of the Food and Agricultural Division, Berlin, wrote on December 6th 1946: 'Senior Commander Law has played an important part. She has cheerfully and loyally worked long hours, often under depressing conditions, and I regard her departure from Germany with considerable misgiving.'

Back in England civilian life awaited with all its uncertainties.

2 Businesswoman

Back in peacetime Britain, Diana set herself to find a job which could make full use of her intelligence and energies.

Daphne Stafford. 'It wasn't easy for her. She had no sort of training, so where was she to go? This is where her drive came out: it had to, to help her family. And once started, she just kept going.'

Faith Porter. 'I remember one job she was offered by an agency was as governess to a small boy in Saudi Arabia! I can't imagine anything less suitable. Anyway, she took a job with the British Council, and later with Shell. She was always very efficient doing her own thing; she couldn't endure being second string. She thought most people in authority should have their heads examined, and often she was dead right!'

Daphne Stafford. 'She had great panache. At the British Council she had a picture of Oxford spires she hung behind her desk: she called it "my university background." '

Anne Handley-Derry. 'There was no doubt that she was extremely capable in her work. When she was made redundant from Shell, she got another high-flown job within a week. I know she was thinking quite seriously of starting up on her own.'

In 1959 Diana joined International Computers and Tabulators Ltd (which in 1969 became International Computers Ltd), first as a personnel officer and later as manager of their Educational Liaison Services.

This was perhaps the most productive period of her business career. Her job involved much travelling, visiting colleges and schools and education authorities to explain to undergraduates, senior students and administrators the potentials of computers in education and society. She designed her own portable displays and organised conferences, such as – in 1966 – a Day Conference on Computer Education in Schools for representatives of local education authorities. She regularly contributed to *Computer Weekly*. She also wrote *Computer Education* for Productivity Progress, and co-operated on *Careers with Computers* for The British Computer Society.

According to Bill Broderick, who met Diana during this period, 'There's no doubt in my mind that the reason the work in educational computing got off the ground and got as far as it has is because of Diana Law.'

W. R. Broderick became interested in the potential of computers after reading maths at university. While teaching at the Royal Liberty School, Romford, he began to concentrate on computer education in schools. This led to the installation of the country's first school computer, which then became the basis of the first local authorities' Educational Computer Centre. Since 1972 he has been Head of the Educational Computer Centre at the London Borough of Havering.

Bill Broderick. 'I first met Diana when I was a young teacher of twenty-two, and concerned to extend the understanding and use of computers in schools. She was an absolute brick. She helped me set up courses for schools: she saw this as the essential way forward.

'I think that initially she was taken on at ICT because they felt that an Educational Liaison Officer was a good thing, and Diana had just the qualities they felt were needed.

She was very personable and sociable and would convey the right impression. At the same time they got something extra they weren't expecting: drive and energy and immense enthusiasm.

'She made things happen. I think at times the company found her rather uncomfortable.

'She was successful because 1) she knew her way around the company; and 2) she had so much energy and enthusiasm and knew how to direct it. She was a perfectionist. She'd get very cross if people fell below par – and she set a high standard for par. Everyone who worked with her worked well and enjoyed it. If she said she would do something, you knew it would get done. She inspired good work and enthusiasm in all those involved with her.'

An excerpt from Diana's curriculum vitae demonstrates how far she had at this point reached in her career.

Is on Staff Management Committee. Member of Institute of Personnel Management and British Computer Society; Chairman of British Computer Society's Working Party on Computer Education in Schools and Computer Careers; on National Association of Youth Clubs (Macalister Brew) Council; and Mathematical Association's Schools and Industry Committee; also on Regional Advisory Council for Technological Education (S.E. Area's) Commercial Committee and the Associated Examining Board's Working Party for a new 'A' Level Syllabus in Computer Science, but is not a mathematician. Is Education and Training Correspondent for *Computer Weekly*.

'ENJOYED SELF!'

As during her army years, though Diana worked hard, she played hard too.

*I like hard work. I don't like sitting about. I like drink-
ing and gambling. I used to drive a combine harvester in
Scotland. Anything like that is great. Housework – horrid!
And I like watching sport too. Athletics. Rugby. Cricket.
Show-jumping! Derby, Grand National always.*

At the same time, there were family crises which she
was called upon to deal with. The sixties, for Diana, were
fruitful but frenetic years.

Daphne Stafford, looking back, says: 'She always had
to do too much. She liked it that way. When I rang her up,
sometimes she'd say, "Hang on, there's someone on the
other line," and she'd leave you hanging on for ages. Sometimes I'd ring off! It could be very irritating, as if she was
the only busy person in the world.

'She worked hard, she played hard, and she drank to
keep going. . . .'

Faith Porter confirms this.

'I can't remember her ever just sitting down and talking.
She flogged herself to keep going. When she came to stay
she couldn't relax. She could *not* relax. "What next?"
she'd say. "What shall we do next?"

'And she was always very closely involved with her
family. Her affections were very much tied to them. She
was their prop and stay. She had a mass of friends, but her
family was the centre.'

Diana says simply:

*Lovely job. Enjoyed self. Going out. Family problems.
Four hours' sleep!*

'A JUMPING BEAN'

Looking back, Diana's friends believe that they detected signs of increasing pressure on her health during the summer and autumn of 1967.

Anne Handley-Derry. 'She had this flat in central London, but it was more of a pied-à-terre. Only one small room, with no real kitchen. She was away practically every week-end, and out most evenings. She'd think nothing of travelling overnight from somewhere and going straight on to lecture first thing in the morning.'

Faith Porter. 'Immediately before her stroke all her friends were saying, "Diana's pushing herself too hard." She was working, rushing back to see her mother, tearing off again. We'd say, "I don't know how she does it." She came to see me just before her stroke. *Very* restless. Like a jumping bean.'

Daphne Stafford. 'That summer before her stroke we went to the races together at Goodwood. She said, "I don't feel well. I've got a temperature." I said, crossly, "You can't simply have a temperature for no reason. You're either ill or you're not."

'I took her off to a tent, and I remember, she was wearing dark glasses; she took them off, and her eyes looked blackened, as though she'd been in a punch-up, dark stains all around them. I didn't think anything of it at the time. I gave her a brandy. Later she seemed fine, and that evening we played tennis with her nephew.

'But I've thought since, perhaps it was a forewarning of her stroke?'

Rosamond Day recalls seeing her only days before.

Rosamond Day first joined the British Council in 1941, and worked for it in various capacities for thirty-three years: in

Liverpool, London, China (where she 'saw history being made' in the changeover to Communism), Brazil and Rome. She first met Diana in 1952, and saw her intermittently from then on between tours of duty. She retired in 1974.

'She came to lunch chez moi on December 2nd, ten days before she had her stroke. The guest Diana came to meet left, and Diana didn't. She stayed on. I thought it rather odd. She was always so organised, always in a hurry. She seemed reluctant to go. I said, "How are you, Di?" And she said, "I've been having a few headaches recently." She asked for aspirins. I've wondered since if those headaches were the first signs of her stroke.'

Diana herself, on that pre-Christmas Wednesday, was sure from the first sign of the warning headache that she was in the process of having a stroke. She says now that she can't explain why she immediately reached this conclusion, but she was never in any doubt at all.

Mid-day, December 13th 1967, was to mark the end of her business career.

3 Stroke

Diana was actually in the middle of a business lunch when her headache started.

Headache, blinding headache. Blinding. Blinding. You can't know. (She puts a hand over her eye and opens and shuts it like blinkers.) *My eyes. . . . They can't see. Personnel officer drive me back to Bowater House. I feel sick. The nurse comes, she says 'bilious.' Two times sick up, but my head is very but very headache.* Please *go to hospital* please. *One hour lost.*
Then comes Marea Hartman, the famous runner. She says no, and sends for an ambulance. She comes with me to hospital.

Marea Hartman competed as a sprint and relay runner from 1936–1955; 'on cinder tracks without running blocks – we had to dig holes in the ground with our little trowels.' During the war she served with the ATS; then worked on the personnel side, first of the Reed Paper Group and then of Bowaters, who allowed her time off to carry on with athletics. She became Olympic Team Manager in 1956 (and has been ever since); also European and Commonwealth Games Team Manager. After 'travelling the world in athletics,' she is now Personnel Consultant with Bowaters. She was awarded first the MBE, and then, in 1979, the CBE.

'I was actually lunching with Diana when it happened.

We'd met through our mutual concern with personnel affairs, at conferences and so on; and partly because we were both interested in sport, and partly through our service experiences, we got on very well together.

'We had in fact met at a nearby German restaurant to discuss the Staff Management Association Conference. When she first began to feel ill, I felt that it could be something serious, and I became more and more convinced. I didn't know what it was. I thought possibly the headaches might be the sign of a coronary. But I felt positive we ought to get her to hospital.'

Then the doctor comes. He says a migraine. All the time the headache, blinding, blinding. My mother comes, and Jacqueline, but I don't notice. The headache . . . frightful.

Then, after some time, I don't know, they take a puncture, in the spine, and they say I have a stroke.

I wanted glasses to keep out the light. My mother and Jacqueline go away and Jacqueline brings the glasses, blue glasses.

Mary Law, Diana's mother, came to London in 1941, after bringing up five children single-handed. She divided her time between her grandchildren, voluntary activities, and painting. Already seventy-eight at the time of Diana's stroke, she was to be 'the key figure,' as Anne Handley-Derry put it, in her recovery. Now ninety, she still holds herself erect and speaks and sings with the true clear voice of her youth, when she won a gold medal for singing at the Dublin Festival 'the year John McCormack got his.'

'It was on December 13th 1967. I had gone over to my married daughter's – Jacqueline's – house at Little Venice. That's where she lived then. We were sitting by the fire – she had coal fires – and the phone rang. Someone said there had been . . . an upset. Diana had suddenly felt ill at her business lunch and had been rushed to hospital. A bad headache, they said.

'I think I knew then. I recognised it. Here we are again. My husband died after a brief and unexpected illness, leaving me alone with five children of four to seventeen. One of my sons was killed in Palestine at the age of twenty-one; he got the Military Cross. I've had so many shocks in my life that this was just another one.

'So it may seem strange, but in a way I felt quite calm as we went, Jacqueline and I, off to the hospital. I remember her husband, David – the actor David Morrell – came back to look after their daughter Angela.

'We saw Diana lying on a trolley. She was obviously in great pain, but the nurse said there was nothing then that could be done.'

Jacqueline Morrell (Lacey) started acting at thirteen, got a scholarship to RADA, and has been an actress ever since. She met her husband in Canada while they were both with the same company, appearing in – among other shows – the first pantomime in North America.

'My mother and I were sitting together when the phone went. We couldn't really make out what was wrong, only that Diana had felt suddenly ill and was now in hospital.

'So I drove there straightaway with my mother. We found Diana there looking dreadful, and I think not really knowing much about what was going on. After a bit I took my mother home. One has to realise that incredible though it sounds now, when later she went on to cope with so much, at the time it started to happen she was already no longer young.

'Later that evening I went back on my own.

'I found Diana more coherent, though she said her head-ache was still blinding, and firing off orders like a shot-gun. She *was* a very busy person. Her diary was full. She did have a lot to tidy up. I quite understood. I thought she sounded lucid and rational. Her instructions came out bang bang bang but they all made sense.

'I went back home and did what she said.

A SUDDEN LOSS OF FUNCTION

'Next day she was transferred to the Atkinson Morley Hospital in Wimbledon.

'The doctor called for me as next-of-kin; I was notified because my mother was already so old. He told me that Diana was having a brain haemorrhage, and that she needed an urgent operation. There was something in an artery, some weakness which had to be tied off, something which meant there was a gradual leakage of blood in the brain; and it had to be done because if it wasn't Diana might die at any moment. Instantly. Without warning.

'No one explained to me that the operation might have other consequences. That Diana might be left paralysed, speechless, and so on. He was a lovely doctor, but he was Belgian, his English wasn't all that good, maybe that was why . . .

'Anyway, of course I said go ahead.

'I feel now, of course I feel I was right, but I did it without really appreciating what might happen. Perhaps for someone not like Diana, without her strength and her outgoingness and her perseverance . . . I don't know. I just think people should be *told*. So that at least they make decisions *knowing* what's involved, not finding out afterwards.

'She had the operation.

'And afterwards she seemed to be making marvellous progress, mending by the day. It seems odd to me now looking back, though I didn't question it at the time, but she wasn't put into intensive care or anything. On the contrary, visitors poured in and out, masses of flowers and ghastly poinsettias, transistor radios, and someone played her a broadcast of some sort of match from somewhere, was it Australia. . . .

'Friends came, and I brought my mother.

'Then one evening David and I were still there visiting, last of all, about three days later, and just about to go. It was a bad winter, 1967–68, very cold. And David made some sort of joke about our car – we had an old Austin then – about how we didn't dare expose it to the winter elements, and Diana said to take her car, her new Triumph. Then she said, and I'll never forget it, that we must have it, because "you do realise, don't you, that the accumulation of the Austin isn't safe?"

'It was such a peculiar thing to say. She'd been sounding so normal, so like her old self, and then suddenly she'd come out with this extraordinary remark.

'We were worried. Even though it was late by the time we got back, David rang the hospital to make sure she was all right.

'They told us that since we'd left Diana had had a major stroke which had left her paralysed and speechless.'

Dr A-M T trained at the Royal Free Hospital School of Medicine after leaving Vienna. She watched the Wolfson Medical Rehabilitation Centre being built, and, after starting her family, went there as its first Registrar, concerned with the rehabilitation of strokes, head injuries and other neurological conditions. She became Deputy Medical Director and remained there for nine years, leaving to join University College Hospital and the Camden Medical Rehabilitation Centre as Consultant in Rehabilitation, with the opportunity to start a stroke unit. She first treated Diana later, in 1968.

'A stroke is an illness, usually of sudden and dramatic onset, due to disease of the blood vessels in or around the brain. This causes death of part of the brain and consequent loss of function – which may be that of speech, vision, movement or feeling at one side of the body – loss of memory, lack of emotional control, or other mental changes. The most common cause is high blood pressure.

'Diana's stroke, however, was unusual in that it was due to a congenital weakness of the blood vessel at the base of the brain. This weakness, or aneurysm as it is called, allowed part of the vessel to balloon out like a weak spot in a tyre under pressure and to burst, causing blood to escape into the brain and so injuring the brain cells. While stress and the aging of blood vessels may have some effect, rupture of an aneurysm may occur in young people and even in children; other people may have similar aneurysms without ever becoming aware of them and without their ever causing any problems.

'Frequently, particularly in younger patients, an operation is carried out to prevent the possibility of further bleeding from the affected vessel; but, unfortunately, though Diana did have this operation, she later had a major stroke which deprived her of speech.'

I don't know the time of the operation. I don't remember. I don't remember the operation much at all. I feel better. No headache.

Then one two three lovely days. Work, work. Visitors come, flocks of visitors. Flowers. Kip brings a transistor. Rugby. The All-Blacks.

New Zealand and Ireland playing. Many people. Then suddenly – two, three days later. At night. The stroke.

Jacqueline Morrell. 'When we went the next day we found Diana in a complete coma. She couldn't move, she couldn't speak. Yet somehow I knew what she meant, even though I can't explain how I managed to understand.

'I remember shortly afterwards, at Christmas-time – it's something you don't forget – hanging Christmas decorations over her bed, and turning the lights full on so I could see what I was doing, and the lights shining down on her and

B

across at all the other poor people in the ward, and she told Angela, my daughter, to leave the ward, that it was too upsetting for her. Well, when I say told, she didn't speak, she indicated, with a movement, but I understood, and Angela went out.'

Gill Hodgson, then on the nursing staff at the Atkinson Morley, remembers Diana from that time; and in particular her friends and family.

Gill Hodgson trained as an SRN at the London Hospital, Whitechapel. After taking a course (for one year at that time) to gain a Diploma in Neurosurgical and Neurological Nursing, she joined the Atkinson Morley in 1967 first as a night sister and then as a junior ward sister.

'Diana came in for life-saving brain surgery. We nursed her through the acute phase, and she then went back to her original hospital. Oddly enough, when she was there I had a call from my brother about her; he was in computers too and knew her slightly. I remember her family and her friends; the way they rallied round, the phone calls, the intelligent questions. It was obvious that Diana must be the same type of person, and I felt that those around her would be better able to cope than many. But otherwise I have no detailed recollection of Diana herself. She was extremely ill. Only one of many patients.'

'VIRTUALLY AN IDIOT'

Mary Law. 'Diana was taken back to the first hospital, and it was there that I met the consultant whose verdict made me so determined to do everything for Diana that was in my power.

'He kept me waiting for three-quarters of an hour, and then he told me: "Your daughter resembles a girl we had here two years ago after a very bad car crash. Today she is virtually an idiot. I'm afraid your daughter's case is hopeless."

'Later I learned that he wasn't a neuro-surgeon but a heart specialist, and not qualified to make such a judgment. I didn't realise this at the time, but what I did know was that it wasn't true.

'I knew my daughter wasn't an idiot. I never for one moment doubted that even though she couldn't communicate she was perfectly conscious of everything that went on. I could tell from her eyes. I wasn't sure what we ought to do next, but I knew we had to find out.'

Jacqueline Morrell. 'I don't know quite what we were expecting, but the consultant's verdict came as a terrible shock. No. I never believed it. If there was any difference between my mother's reaction and my own, I think I'd say that my mother felt *convinced* that one day my sister would be just as she was, while I wasn't quite so certain in my mind. Oh, I knew she wasn't an idiot, I could tell she was all there inside, but I could see something drastic had happened. I didn't know how much recovery we could really hope for.'

Marea Hartman. 'When I first saw her after her stroke you couldn't help wondering if she'd ever make it. But I had the example of my mother. During the war doctors had told her she'd never walk again – she had a fractured skull, a war injury – but she *did*. She not only walked, she could even skip! At the age of sixty-three. I saw then what will-power could do, and I told Diana about her.

'I didn't doubt her courage. I knew she could understand. But still – she couldn't say much; well, nothing at all, apart from these grunting noises.'

The next weeks remain for Diana as a confused and anguished memory of despair, helplessness and frustration.

It was the most terrifying experience of her life. Doctors and nurses would consult about her over her head as though she didn't exist. Lying there totally unable to communicate her wishes and emotions except with her eyes, she vowed that if she recovered, *when* she recovered, she would dedicate the rest of her life to all those similarly afflicted.

Very lot of people come. Very lot of people visit me, but I can't speak. And I . . . I like talking! Very *frustrating. I want something, I know what, but nurses too busy. Now much better. Then* nothing. *All treated me like an idiot. Mother and Jacqueline, lots of time spend half an hour trying to get one thing across. Had* Times, *looked at births and marriage, but perhaps not read it! Funny.*

Diana's insecurity and frustration were compounded by the fact that no one, at any point during this period immediately after her stroke, explained to her *why* she could suddenly no longer find the words to speak; why, almost overnight, the power to communicate had been snatched from her. As she was to put it some years later: 'Doctors and nurses . . . very kind. But . . . loopy, you know. Loopy.'

Her friends' reactions varied, but with few exceptions they rallied round to give her every possible encouragement. A touching scribbled note from this time begs: 'DIANA IS DELIGHTED AND TOUCHED BY YOUR COMING TO SEE HER BUT WILL YOU PLEASE NOT STAY FOR MORE THAN TEN MINUTES.'

Anne Handley-Derry. 'That December when she got her stroke, I didn't have a Christmas card from her. I wasn't bothered, I merely thought I'd hear from her soon. Then I ran into a friend who told me what had happened.

'I went to see her in the hospital – back in the first one, after her operation, after her stroke proper.

'I found her in the terminal geriatric ward. It was a shock. Her young face among all those dear old things at the end of their lives. The next time I went she was out in another ward. She couldn't say a thing, except a sort of "ooh-hooh!" noise, but she was surrounded by flowers and people and I knew she knew what was going on. I talked to her about Germany, her job at ICT. . . . I told her, "We'll be laughing at this together before too long." '

Daphne Stafford. 'When I heard of her stroke, I was very worried about what I might find.

'My brother had already been to see her in the Atkinson Morley, after her first stroke and before her second. Diana seemed worried and tense, she'd called someone from her office and was there dictating work . . .

'Anyway, when I went to see her back in the hospital after her operation I was surprised at her liveliness. We laughed together, we had a really jolly evening. I came back vastly cheered. I felt there was very little handicap. When I went back on the second occasion, I felt she had slipped back in her speech. I realised then how little in fact she had said before. I suppose it was because we felt the same way, laughed at the same things . . .'

Rosamond Day. 'To start with, only her family were allowed to visit Diana. At the time of her second haemorrhage, I was due to leave London to go north for Christmas. So it was only after I returned, and after the operation, that I could visit her for the first time after her stroke. She smiled, and seemed much better. I went again a week later, and gave her a manicure. I knew she was ill, but I didn't question *why*. I just accepted it. She could always get across to her mother what she was thinking.'

'MUCH HELP'

Gradually, with painful slowness, Diana began to improve, beginning with a move from the geriatric ward –

in which she had been placed on her return – and from the ward sister who insisted on treating her like an infant, and into another ward with a 'lovely sister' who offered endless encouragement to her and her relatives.

Her mother and sister came every day; bit by bit problems were met and overcome.

Jacqueline Morrell. 'Diana stayed on in the hospital for another three months. I gave up working. Altogether I gave up work for a year, so I could be free to drive my mother down and see Diana myself. Mostly I'd go over in the mornings and then come back and take my mother in the afternoons.'

Mary Law. 'On the whole they were very good to her in hospital. To start with there were problems. The first sister she had seemed inefficient and casual. There were little things. Her teeth weren't washed at night. And – it seems extraordinary, but of course the time I'm talking about was nearly twelve years ago now – nobody attended to her physical needs during the night, so she was constantly having a wet bed. They thought she was incontinent, but it wasn't that. There was just no way she could communicate that she wanted a bed-pan. When at first I asked why she couldn't have a buzzer she could just press, they said because all the other patients would want one too!

'Finally, that was sorted out, and in small practical ways things got better.'

Diana, with a grin, endorses the essential.

Had Guinness twice a day lunch and dinner! My mother and Jacqueline bring it. Many visitors. Much help.

Physically, thanks to the physiotherapy and occupational

therapy, she began to make progress. Gradually she learnt to walk again, with the help of a tripod.

Jacqueline Morrell. 'She began to stand and move and dress herself. The occupational therapist rang me one day to say, "You just must come and see Diana getting dressed! I'm amazed at the way she's getting on."

'So I went down – I caught the bus, the car had given up the ghost by then– and I watched her getting dressed, sitting on the bed, and somehow putting on everything with one hand. It was incredibly moving. It sounds strange, perhaps, but it was. I nearly cried. To watch the perseverance, the determination.'

OT wonderful in this hospital. I dress myself. This woman help me. Two hours and a half! Tired out. Lunch. Then undress.

'TONIGHT AND TONIGHT AND TONIGHT'
The lack of speech, however, remained – as it was to remain for months and years – as an ever-present, insurmountable barrier. No one, either on the medical staff or among her family and friends, seemed to know what steps to take.

Jacqueline Morrell. 'Diana still couldn't speak. I used to try to help her. I suppose you could say I was her very first speech therapist! They were good to me at the hospital. They used to give me a little room so we could be alone together. I'd try to get her to say things like "bacon and eggs," " whisky and soda," "gin and tonic." I thought that was very Diana, "gin and tonic."

'She didn't speak, but I could tell from her eyes that she understood. I felt that we were on the same wavelength.'

Diana had also, very briefly, some sessions of 'speech therapy' paid for by BUPA, but which were, she says firmly, no more than elocution. She remained for weeks almost totally without speech.

Then, almost imperceptibly, the first intimations began to emerge.

Jacqueline Morrell. 'It seems strange I don't remember exactly when it was; but she started to speak. She had one word. "Tonight." It meant anything and everything. She used it all the time. I was never in any doubt as to what she intended it to mean.'

Nancy Esterson, the 'lovely sister' who proved such a mainstay to the Law family, explains how Diana's lack of speech appeared at the time.

Nancy Esterson trained as an SRN after taking a degree in English. She was a Medical Ward sister when she first met Diana; she has since worked at Charing Cross, then Edgware General Hospital, and is now Divisional Nursing Officer at St Bartholomew's.

'I must say right away that the holes in the system at that time have since become far more apparent to me. I know more about strokes now. I certainly didn't appreciate then the necessity of speech therapy. I'd have stamped my foot much harder on behalf of my patients if I had.

'I'd had several other stroke patients to care for, but they'd mostly been much older. Diana's comparative youth was a shocking feature; though I never saw her when she was in the most critical state – she'd been a patient for some weeks before I was appointed sister on her ward. I knew from her files what sort of background she'd had, and I could tell from her general appearance – she was very alert – that she understood.

'She was a mass of frustration. Her only speech at that time was "Tonight and tonight *and* tonight and . . . tonight *and and* tonight." She tried to speak using just those words with different ways of emphasis.'

'The student nurses were baffled. So was I! They all tried hard to understand but all of them were in awe of her because she looked like someone in command. No matter how we tried I never got another dicky bird out of her.

'I tried to have twenty minutes' conversation with her every day. Very egocentric – I just chattered on about me and my family. One is always a bit self-conscious when you know someone can't reply, but I felt much less so with Diana, because I knew it all went in. I was sure she understood. She's told me since that she appreciated it, because she felt there were people who simply believed she was an idiot.

'I still have paroxysms of guilt whenever I think of her. Perhaps I didn't communicate adequately to my staff? Perhaps there was a shortfall in summoning para-medical help? Looking back, I probably didn't pull out all the stops. I would do more now.

'I felt that Diana's frustration became determination. She recognised that frustration didn't bring rewards, and turned her mind and energies to a course which would.'

THE NEXT STEP
Diana's family and friends felt helpless.

Mary Law. 'I could imagine how frustrating it must be for someone like Diana not to be able to speak, but it was difficult to know where to go for help. Nobody discussed this with us. Nobody explained what had happened, what these speech difficulties were. There was no speech therapist at the hospital. I suppose we'd heard of speech therapy, but I think like a lot of people we thought of it as being a bit like chiropody, instead of the vital service it ought to be.'

Jacqueline Morrell. 'We'd been told that probably the best place for someone like Diana to be was the Wolfson Medical Rehabilitation Centre in Wimbledon.

'We met with tremendous opposition. I think at that time people, even medical people, knew very little about strokes. The consultant's report had been so damning, and the Wolfson weren't keen on taking someone who appeared to have so little long-term prospects.

'So I set about writing letters. I wrote letters to anyone I thought would listen, anyone I thought might help. Isaac Wolfson, Rex Cohen – the head of Selfridge's – people she'd known in the army.

'At about the same time, Diana started to switch from "tonight" to "other people."

'I don't know why, but this baffled me. I couldn't tell what she meant any more. She'd say "other people," in this very accusing voice, and I just didn't know. It was disturbing.

'Anyway, in the end the Wolfson decided to take her.

'It was a terrible time. David and I drove her over – that's to say, I drove, because David was beginning to feel the effects of his illness – and we took her there and left her, entirely on her own, unable to speak or communicate, all alone with all these desperately disabled people.

'Outside I cried for half an hour in the car. I cried and cried and couldn't stop.

'She looked so alone.'

4 Towards speech at the Wolfson

Dr A-M T. 'Diana was first admitted to the Wolfson on 3 March 1968, and remained until 31 May.

'She had little speech recovery and severe hemiplegia. She had no function in the right arm, but was walking reasonably well with a tripod. She was not depressed*; in fact she seemed slightly euphoric. She gave the impression that she understood well, but later it was wondered whether she did in fact understand so well, or whether it might be an illusion due to her general responsiveness. She had no idea of numbers, and very little writing, but she concentrated well in psychological tests.'

Diana shared a room with a very brave but greatly handicapped woman who was totally confined to her bed. It seemed a kind of irony to her; to see two women together one of whom could move but couldn't speak, the other who could speak but couldn't move.

Her days here were full and very strenuous, alternating between therapy, periods of hard physical activity, and rest.

They make me this calliper. Before that, I have to wear always woolly boots. During the day I'm happy there. And the Guinness is free!

* Throughout this book, the words 'depression' and 'depressed' are used in their colloquial and not clinical sense.

Best of all, for the very first time, Diana met someone who understood her lack of speech, explained to her how it had happened, and set her on the road to recovery: her first speech therapist, Michael Jackson.

Years later, in the prize-winning essay she wrote with her speech therapist, Joan Ellams*, she summed up her feelings at this stage of her stroke.

It was at this time that I realised that not only could I not talk – I could not read or write either – what a catastrophe! I could not speak, although my tongue worked perfectly well and I knew what I wanted to say. I could not always fully understand what people said to me, although I was not the slightest deaf; I could not read, although I could see the words quite clearly on the page – they just had no meaning; I could not write, although by this time I had learnt to use a pencil with my left hand – I could in fact copy-write quite beautifully. As with my speech: I knew what I wanted to write but I could not find the words, and even when I could I could not spell them. . . .

Diana recognises that Michael Jackson, not only through his professional dedication, but by his personal understanding, was of immense importance in her fight back to independence.

Michael Jackson trained in speech therapy at the Central School. He went first to work with mentally-handicapped children and adults at Botleys Park, Chertsey, and then with neurological patients at the Wolfson; in this way 'gaining perception of language at both ends – from, the study of non-emergent language to that of language which has receded.' He then joined the staff at the Oldrey-Fleming School of Speech Therapy in Hampstead, and after its amalgamation with the

* See page 151

West End Hospital Speech Therapy Training School joined the new combined National Hospitals College of Speech Sciences. Here he lectures on second-year studies while continuing his clinical work at the Royal Free and, most recently, Adult Training Centres.

'When I first met Diana at the Wolfson there was no clinical difference at all between her and many many other patients. She was unusually young to have had a stroke at all, but otherwise she was a classic case. It was severe, and bad because it occurred in her *left* cerebral hemisphere and therefore affected her *right* leg and *right* hand. This was doubly unfortunate as she was by nature a right-handed person and – like practically all right-handers as well as many left-handers* – had a major speech coding centre located in the left cerebral hemisphere.

'Diana had all of this. The only words she had were "It's madness! It's wonderful! My dear!" though she managed to make them convey a great deal.

'I've made short broadcast recordings a few times with Diana, and I remember once she broke down completely when she was describing her feelings just after her stroke. It was concern for others though, and not for herself. She was describing her feelings of aloneness and helplessness, the way people don't understand that even though the affected person may not respond, the inner core is still there; the way people speak over them and to them as though they don't exist.

'I've seen some dreadful things, though, obviously (also some wonderful ones as well). I've seen nurses, and I mean experienced nurses, not ones in training, behave in a way you wouldn't believe. The sort of thing like, "Oh, Mr Johnson, aren't we a naughty boy, we didn't finish up our carrots," to a man who only days before might have been at the top of his job or profession. Diana understood very

* See also page 156

well all the anger and anguish this kind of attitude can cause. This is one of the things, I'm sure, which spurred her on.

FIRST STAGES

'I used to give her individual therapy every day; in addition she had group therapy.

'We started at a very elementary level. The first stage is to try to establish what understanding there is. Where there are difficulties, these may be caused by problems with hearing – which wasn't true of Diana – or through two different kinds of incomprehension: the first caused by lack of memory (the patient can't retain the significance of more than a very few words at a time) or complete unintelligibility (the words mean no more to the patient than Japanese to a monolingual English-speaking person).

'With Diana her understanding problems were caused by the memory thing. So I concentrated on short phrases, short instructions. Everything was very simple, very basic.

'Then we did a lot of vocabulary work. Again, very simple. We would look at pictures. I would say, "Show me the table. Which is the cup?"

'All your patients are different. Anything may happen. You can show a picture of a cup, and the patient may say "drink." The code-word is lost, but the connection is there in the mind. With some patients the picture itself means nothing. They can't relate to the two-dimensional representation. They have to see the object itself. In general we prefer to use pictures, simply because of the practical difficulty of assembling a whole lot of objects, but with some patients the presence of actual things is the only way forward. Diana could cope with pictures, though, right from the beginning.

'She always worked extremely hard, even when her concentration was poor. She would watch my lip movements, and study the expression on my face. It's always important when speaking to a stroke patient to look directly, speak clearly, and not, for example, hide your mouth by putting your hand in front of it. Some patients rely a lot on gesture to convey their meaning, but Diana never did. Some people in some cultures (or groups within cultures) use a lot of gesture, but Diana is not a gesture person – which makes the recovery of actual speech even more important.

'We then progressed to reading single words, and even to attempting to write. This means writing with the left hand, which is very difficult mechanically. There's not only the problem of recalling the word and the shape of the word, but the physical problem of outlining this shape on the paper.

'We didn't do any syntax at this time. Diana wasn't ready for it. I concentrated on vocabulary, figure work, and lots of encouragement. We have to think of the *individual* patient. What that patient was like, what that patient will need in the future. Diana needed speech, reading, writing, calculation – especially money calculation. She would need to be able to handle her own finances, so we did simple mathematical work. 2 + 2 – that sort of thing.

'Group therapy gave her the opportunity to practise what had been started in individual therapy. We had two groups at that time. Diana was in the elementary one, called euphemistically "speech games". It was very small – never more than three patients at once. Any more, and you can't give them the individual attention they need.

'We helped them to tackle any kind of simple speech puzzles – matching words on cards, written words to pictures, pairing objects, picking out sequences and so on. The higher class of course went on to more elaborate exercises, but Diana couldn't yet tackle anything like that.

'In fact, by the time she left us she hadn't advanced very far. It's a slow business, recovering speech, and there's no steady progress. It can be very disheartening, especially for relatives who only see the patient at intervals. I'd like to emphasise that it's not like learning a foreign language, where a word once learnt stays learnt – or on the whole it does. For dysphasics, a word can be recaptured and then lost again, so that the patient can seem to go backwards rather than forwards.

HOW PERSONALITY COUNTS

'But I always told Diana, as I tell all my patients, that she *would* get better, that her speech *would* improve, that a stroke was not a complete barrier, that in spite of all her disabilities great things could still be done. I think Diana has successfully proved that this can be so. Of course she always had the support of a marvellous family and, even in the very early days, immense determination.

'One of the main factors influencing recovery is the premorbid personality. After a stroke a personality change tends to be one of degree rather than of type – people become more what they already were. I hadn't known Diana before, but I suspect she always was a determined forceful person who would make up her mind what her goal would be, and then drive straight ahead for it. You could see this determination driving her right from the time I first met her. She has also always been able to be objective about herself – this is comparatively rare in my experience. She is able to say of herself: "I have changed in this way and that."

'There's one other quality in Diana which is perhaps exceptional.

'She has never, because what she has is not as good as what she had, allowed herself to give up. This is rare for a person like her with her background and education. We therapists used to think that the educated person must be the most satisfying to treat, because they have so many interests, so many hooks to make contact, to draw out the

language. They're not. Oh, they can be stimulating for the
therapist, but they can be absolute hell to rehabilitate. High-
powered people are often demanding and dissatisfied. They
want to get back to what they were. Then, because what
they achieve is never good enough, they give up. Diana
has never been like that. She's been demanding, very
demanding, but she has never given up. She found people
to push her too, and she's just carried on.

'People's recovery is not only dependent on their personality, and on other basic factors such as age, general health,
site of the lesion, their environment, but on the life they
led and the life they see as potential: they also improve to
some extent in the way that they themselves see as important.

'I often think of Diana and Colonel "Bloody Hell"
Martin together. They met at the Wolfson and then went
to Osborne House on the Isle of Wight* at the same time,
and became good friends. They were both intelligent, communicating people, they both suffered a disabling stroke,
but they recovered in different ways. The Colonel had led a
very vigorous life, rode to hounds and so on. He had no
obvious limb impairment, but he didn't improve much in
his expressive speech at all (as opposed to his understanding, which was always good). He just had these two magnificent cavalry expressions: "Bloody Hell!" and "God's
teeth!" He was completely mobile, got around London
without any difficulty.

'The Colonel's reaction, when things went wrong, was
quite different from Diana's. It was anger. He would hit
out antagonistically at things – metaphorically I mean –
and then draw back and smash headlong at the problem
again, without pausing to consider. Diana's was more of
distress. She would chisel away gradually at things, plug-
ging away to try to overcome the problem.

'In the end he died of cancer. I must admit I never told

* See page 129

Diana at the time, and on one occasion feigned a lack of knowledge as to what had become of him after our last chance meeting in London. I did this to protect her, but – as I look back at it now – I can see that this was unnecessary. Diana has such great reserves of spiritual strength that she is well able to cope.

'This is another problem with dysphasics. How much do you tell them? They tend to be more emotionally labile. Because they become sometimes disproportionately upset, one begins to censor the information one gives them. It's natural to feel that someone who has already suffered so much should, as far as possible, be spared further suffering, but then naturally one runs the risk of over-protecting, of not treating them as independent adults, and the perceptive patient will, in the long run, become aware that certain things are being withheld, and become resentful.

'It's hard, especially for relatives, to find the balance. Most oscillate between different states of mind; and the patient's condition is not static. That's one of the reasons adult centres are good, because it gives the therapist more chance to meet the relatives and help both them and their relationship with the patients.

'It can also help us to establish the best avenue of approach; because not all dysphasics want to work. They can be very ambivalent. Some are single-minded like Diana. Others would like to make an effort, but keep putting it off; they get diverted. Others simply give up. Between us – the relatives, the patients, the therapists – we can try to decide what methods are the most likely to produce results.

'Another great source of strength for Diana has been her religious faith. As an observer, it seems to me that she has never wavered. Deep down she has always had absolute certainty.

'I always remember her too for her social awareness – something which stroke patients often lose to a certain degree. There was one occasion when Diana came back to the Wolfson on a visit, not as a patient, not long after she'd left. Her speech was still very limited. She came and saw me and a colleague and we chatted together and there were lots of "My dear! My dear!" And then it was 2 p.m., and it was really time for my colleague and me to go and start work, but we neither of us quite knew how to get away. There was no one around, and it seemed rude just to go off and abandon her on her own in the corridor. So we stayed on five minutes more, chatting away; and Diana became aware of the situation. She still had virtually no speech to communicate what she felt. I shall aways remember: she flung out her arms wide and embraced us both, and said: "Well, my dears!"

'It was quite obvious what she meant. She felt the implications of the moment, she had the delicacy to deal with it, and she used the speech that she had to cope in her own particular way. It ended any possible feeling of awkwardness.'

MAKING PROGRESS

Diana's medical notes document her achievements during these months.

Dr A-M T. 'By the beginning of April her speech was improving and new words were coming. She had difficulties reading aloud, but she could read silently and answer multiple choice questions. She couldn't spell, but could copy words.

'She then became very frustrated with her lack of communication: we think this is when the understanding of her position suddenly came home to her. Group therapy was added to her individual speech therapy. She progressed well, and by the end of April she could do dictation if the words were spelt.

'Physically too she improved, though she had a fit at the

end of March, which had no permanent effects. Her walking progressed well. We tried to help her get rid of her calliper, but it made her too tired. We got her a new one, which made a difference.

'By the end of May she could raise her right arm to her mouth, but had little movement in her hand. She could walk well with a stick, overcome small obstacles, stand for twenty minutes, and carry something small. She was personally independent (i.e. she could bath herself etc. with the right aids), and cope with ordinary household activities. She had done some shopping under supervision, and had gone on public transport, but without being too happy about it. Her speech suffered greatly under stress, and she had little confidence in her ability to communicate.'

During these weeks Diana's friends and family continued to rally round her. Daphne Stafford remembers taking her out for drives; Marea Hartman and her colleagues took her in the evening to a nearby pub on Wimbledon Common, and once to a restaurant: 'But it had to be somewhere without stairs. She couldn't manage those. That's why the pub was easier for her.' Marea also remembers:

'It was a great boost to her when she found she could open a bottle again! It was in the Wolfson; a bottle of whisky. It was perfectly legitimate, we asked first – but the pleasure on her face when she found she could manage it again! She loves offering hospitality, and it meant a lot to her to be able to offer a drink herself.'

I'm happy there. I'm making progress. Only in the evenings no social life. And the week-ends – deadly! But then Jacqueline and David drive over and pick me up.

Jacqueline and her husband fetched her most week-ends, together with her four pillows and three blankets and two large suitcases. Her family began to see the first real signs of improvement.

Then, suddenly – as Diana sees it – it was time to leave.

5　Interim

One minute I'm happy. Then suddenly I have to go. I'm very sad. I must say this. People should have warning. More warning. At least two weeks. Or it's a shock.

Jacqueline Morrell. 'When Diana was discharged it was a Bank Holiday weekend. We had to try at short notice and over the holiday to get safety bars fitted in our flat; by the bath and round the walls and so on. It turned out to be the most tremendous battle. We rang the Health Service, and the Social Security people came round and asked us about our income. They seemed much more concerned about who was paying and how much it was than about the practical problem of getting it done and the need to get it done quickly for Diana's actual safety. Somehow we managed to get hold of a man and in the end got it all fixed. It was all done privately and we paid for it ourselves.

'And Diana moved in.

'The idea at that time was that she would stay with us and my mother alternately, a few weeks or months at a time. David gave up his writing-room for her sitting-room, and our spare room became her bedroom. We thought this would give us all a degree of privacy and independence.

'We meant it for the best, but I can see now that it was a great mistake. What she needed most of all was to be with people, living with them and listening to them and trying to communicate, and not feel shut away. I don't say it mightn't have suited someone else, but it was all wrong for Diana.

'Not that I want you to get the idea that we simply left her alone. David especially was marvellous. He was much better than I was at coping to start with. He worked in television, so luckily we had different hours. They spent ages playing dominoes and cards together. When David died a few years later, Diana wrote me a marvellous letter through a scribe.

' "I have felt very much that I wanted to express to you more adequately than my words (speech) can do, how very sad I was at David's death.

' "I have always had a great fondness for David and have appreciated so much his kindness to me, especially when I was in hospital and in the early days of my recovery. He was helpful in encouraging me to have confidence for walking out in the street again. . . .

' "I shall always remember our mutual love of black pudding, and the pleasure we had when playing card games together. David thoughtfully gave me the Lone Arm card holder which he had found. . . ."

'(Then, in Diana's own hand : –)'
' "good luck, god bless, good health, much love   Di."

'In spite of our intentions, though, at the time the balance was wrong.

'Anyway, after a few weeks my agent rang me up and told me I'd had an offer to play at the Belgrade in Coventry. I hadn't acted for a year. My agent told me that I couldn't go on refusing work if I actually wanted to stay in the theatre at all. He said if I turned this offer down he would take my name off his books, and as far as he was concerned I'd be finished.

'So I took the job. It wasn't easy. I remember it was very

cold again, and then there was a rail strike. . . . For three weeks David looked after Diana on his own, but it simply couldn't go on like that, especially as David's own health was deteriorating.

'And Diana went back to the room she still has in my mother's flat.

'Later she used her own flat from time to time during the day, and she often visited us for weekends over the next six months until David became really ill, but that small room was her home from then on.'

6   From the depths

The next six-month period – from July to December 1968 – was perhaps the nadir for both Diana and her mother. As her friend Rosamond Day put it: 'Diana went down to the depths herself. Only her courage and persistence – and her family closing round her – pulled her out of it.'

Mary Law. 'Those months between the Wolfson and the Camden were, I think, the worst of all. I had some guidance from Diana's speech therapists, but otherwise I was on my own. All the time, then and afterwards, I would be talking to her. I'd talk and talk. I took no notice if she didn't speak or didn't seem to respond. I simply went on talking. Or I'd say things like "What's that? It's a table," and go on repeating it; only I couldn't do that for too long because Diana tired very quickly.

'I couldn't have gone on except that I never had any doubt that even when she seemed least responsive she was still there listening. But yes, it was very hard. It was the hopelessness of it that was the worst. And the silence. The silence all around me all the time. I found it very hard to cope. When I began to feel really desperate I would turn away from her and towards the wall and pull the most awful grimaces.

'It's not like teaching a child. With this – there is always sorrow there. The contrast with what used to be.

'Saturdays and Sundays were nightmares. Our neighbours were very kind, but they didn't understand. They would call on us and talk to me but not to her. Her friends came, of course, but even the best of friends can't come all the time.

'But Diana was very brave. All this time I never once heard her complain.'

It was not a time of total dejection. Diana went for a few weeks to Roehampton Hospital, and this proved a welcome break.

Very successful. Not speech therapy but OT and walking and all that.

Daphne Stafford. 'She was in an enormous ward, sort of Boer War-ish, a brain-cum-geriatrics ward I think, lines of beds on each side. I thought, how can she bear it? But she got on terribly well, had everyone completely under her thumb. She thoroughly enjoyed it there.'

The ups however were too often followed by downs. Even her first visit to the King Edward VII's Convalescent Home at Osborne*, which was later to give her so much happiness, upset her.

Daphne Stafford. 'She went to Osborne for the first time from Roehampton. It was a dead failure. She kept ringing me up in tears, and ringing Jacqueline too. I believe it was because Osborne brought home to her the fact that at that time she couldn't keep up with the intellectual level of the people she met there.

'Some time later she went to two other convalescent homes with her mother. One was a complete failure too.

* See page 129

She rang me up and asked me to come over to see her. I said it was too far, and I'd call when she got back to London. Then I felt there was something not right, and fifteen minutes later I rang back. Her mother answered, and said: "Thank heavens. She's been crying ever since you rang off." I think the reason that time was that there were mainly geriatric patients there, and no one at all she could have a real conversation with.'

However, during this period of what must sometimes have felt to Diana like complete stagnation, there appeared two gleams of light.

The first was the possibility of her admission to the Camden Medical Rehabilitation Centre.

Jacqueline Morrell. 'Almost as soon as she moved out of the Wolfson we began to make great efforts to get her into the Camden Rehabilitation Centre. We'd heard a lot about it, and we were sure it was the right place for her. We felt strongly that after all the work Diana had been doing at the Wolfson she couldn't just stop at home and let it all slip away. The Wolfson had originally suggested the Centre, but to start with Camden turned her down – just as the Wolfson had, and I think for the same reason: because at that time anyhow they preferred shorter-term patients and ones who they felt had a more hopeful future. We kept on working away at them; it took quite a while, but in the end they agreed.'

The second was her meeting with Joan Ellams: who, says Jacqueline, 'was perhaps more than anyone else the one who transformed Diana's life.'

Joan Ellams trained for three years at the West End Hospitals

School for Speech Therapy (now the National College of Speech Sciences), and then worked at Liverpool for eighteen months with both children and adults. She came to the CMRC in 1965 'almost by accident,' after a friend she had trained with had had to leave and suggested she might be interested. She gave it a try, liked it, was accepted, and has been there ever since.

'I first met Diana in June 1968. It was arranged through her sister, at the time she was staying with Jacqueline during the week and spending the week-ends with her mother.

'She was very bright – I could see that from the expression in her eyes. She still has that brightness, that force; and you could see it even then. But she was very depressed. She had limited understanding and virtually no speech.

'I assessed her on June 6th, using *Examining for aphasia*, by Jon Eisenson. (Aphasia is complete lack of language; dysphasia is partial lack of language.) From the results of the test I concluded that Diana was "a woman of very high intelligence who has a severe predominantly executive dysphasia with some receptive loss . . . more marked for the written word than the spoken word." She had very little spontaneous speech: "Yes;" "But;" "It's wonderful;" "It's madness;" but these phrases were all used appropriately. She had moderate dyslexia and marked dysgraphia: that is, she had considerable difficulty in reading and very great difficulty in writing. I added at the time: "The patient is depressed but tries hard to hide it."

'I began to see her twice a week: once at Jacqueline's and once at her mother's. (BUPA contributed to the cost.) In addition, David brought her once a week by taxi to the Rehabilitation Centre to join in a group speech therapy session.'

This difficult period of Diana's life came to an end on January 14th 1969, just over a year after her initial stroke, when she joined the CMRC as a full-time patient.

It was to prove a major turning-point in her recovery.

7   The Camden Medical Rehabilitation Centre

At Camden Medical Re-ha-bi-li-ta-tion Centre I work very, very hard. I like it enormously. Individual speech therapy once a day, group speech therapy once a day, gymnasium, remedial exercises, occupational therapy, writing – I'm not any good! A lot of exercises. Fit ones standing up, not fit ones sitting down, swinging arms, legs and so on for half an hour. Very good! I'm very happy!

With her customary ability to get across the essential, Diana sums up a year's intense activities in a few precise words.

To understand more fully how this Centre functions, and how patients like Diana are taught and urged and coaxed back towards recovery and a fuller life, listen to Wenona Keane as she escorts a party of visitors around.

Wenona Keane worked for United Dairies during the war, then trained at the London School of Occupational Therapy. She taught there following her first OT job at Bromley Hospital, and joined CMRC in 1955, where she has been ever since. She is now their Rehabilitation/Administrative Officer.

'The Camden Medical Rehabilitation Centre was founded in 1954, at the inspiration of Dr C.J.S.O'Malley, who had pioneered rehabilitation work during the war. After the treatment he initiated, 80 per cent of the badly injured air-crews he helped went back to full flying duties. When the war was over he opened Garston Manor, a residential centre, to make available the same techniques for civilians.

'It was then suggested that a non-residential centre might make good sense. It would be more economical to run; it would be better psychologically for patients to be based in their own homes; it would help to hasten their return to normal life.

'Accordingly, in 1954 the CMRC opened its doors to a full staff and four patients, who must have enjoyed the most intensive therapy ever! Within a very short time, the intake of patients built up to eighty. (This is the absolute maximum; seventy-five is more comfortable.) We feel that this is the largest number compatible with individual care. With more people, there would be a risk that both staff and patients would not be able to know each other well.

'The original aim of the Centre, and which still remains a basic consideration, was to rehabilitate the patients to enable them to return to work as quickly as possible. This gives them a goal; restores self-confidence; provides motivation which helps them to work at their own recovery. Some patients will return to their original work. Others will find alternative work, which may or may not be with their previous employers. Yet others will go for re-training, at a government centre or a special college for disabled people. Some, unfortunately, will never return to any form of work: for them what is sought is an improvement in the quality of life, and they will go under the care of the Social Services.

'Treatment at the Centre means five-day attendance for six hours a day. It's not suitable for small children, who would find the regime too exhausting, but apart from that restriction patients are from any age from fourteen upwards. There's no upper age limit: the oldest patient so far has been ninety-three. Rehabilitation may enable older people to lead a more independent life, and in turn take some of the pressure off involved relatives.

'Patients come to the CMRC from three sources. 80 per cent are referred by hospitals, not only locally but further afield; the only qualification is that patients should not have more than two hours' travelling a day, as we feel that the fatigue caused by longer journeys would out-weigh any benefits. 15 per cent are referred by GPs; mainly local. The other 5 per cent come through Industrial Medical Officers, doctors attached to large factories, foundries, mines, the Port of London Authority, and so on.

'98 per cent of those referred are accepted. The only qualification is that rehabilitation must be a practicable possibility. The only ones turned down – very reluctantly – are those with extremely severe multiple disabilities or those who have been confined to a bed or wheelchair so long that rehabilitation can no longer be considered possible. As Dr S. once wrote in a letter to an over-optimistic doctor, "Rehabilitation should not be confused with resurrection."

'There is and can be no compulsion on patients to attend, but absenteeism is extremely low. With allowances made for genuine absence (for illness or attendance at hospitals), average daily attendance is 98 per cent.

'Approximately 50 per cent come under their own steam. 50 per cent are brought by ambulance or car service.

'Admissions are always made on either Monday or Tuesday. Experience has shown that most patients get stiff – *very* stiff! – on the second or third day of treatment. By the weekend this has begun to wear off, the patient begins to feel the possibility of improvement, and can be relied upon to return the following Monday. End-of-the-week admissions, in former days, resulted in a weekend's creaking and groaning after the initial treatment, and too often a failure to re-submit themselves to more of the same the following Monday. Beginning-of-the-week admissions have changed all this.

'The same thinking lies behind the regular discharge on Fridays. Those who are going back to work thus have a normal weekend at home, followed by straight-back-to-work the following Monday. In the past, leaving too long a gap between discharge and the start at work led to too much time for brooding and dreading the inevitable plunge back into a working life after what might have been a long interval.

THE PROGRAMME

'For all new patients the initial programme is the same.

'They're warmly greeted, and given a pair of shorts (or a short skirt) and a shirt which will be their everyday uniform in the Centre. This is for three reasons: first, it's important for the staff to be able to see exactly how a limb is functioning; second, because a lot of messy work is done in occupational therapy, and this is a simple way to protect patients' home-going clothes; and third, because it helps to level out social differences between all those who attend the Centre. All patients are there for similar reasons, all can give support and inspiration to others: money and dress should not create barriers.

'The first staff member patients talk to is the social worker. In this way immediate personal problems can be tackled. This is essential. Any worries – over money or children or even over who's going to do the shopping – can prevent treatment from being effective.

'Next they see the Sister to be weighed and measured and to discuss any medicines being currently taken.

'After this they visit the doctor for a full medical check-up and a review of their medical history.

'Last of all the doctor and I get together to plan individual programmes for each patient, which will go on being modified to match progress all the time they remain at the Centre.

'We then take the patients on a tour to introduce them

C

to each department.The programme-planning must fit the patients' needs – we don't expect them to fit in to a highly-structured regime. We're small enough, and we have a large enough staff, to be able to maintain this individual care.

'Each day lasts from 9.30–4.30, split into seven forty-minute periods: four in the morning, with a break for tea and a snack, then lunch, then three periods with tea and biscuits. The kitchen and canteen staff form a vital part of our team. Often they can provide an illuminating side-light on a patient's condition.

REMEDIAL GYMNASTICS

'Both morning and afternoon sessions start with a warm-ing-up period to music. The patients are divided into *standing*, *sitters*, and *slow-sitters*; all get thirty minutes' exercise. The only difference between sitters and slow-sitters is that the slow ones do the same exercises but take two beats of music for each movement instead of one.

'Our aim is to encourage patients to use their whole bodies. We want to restore their confidence by helping them to get as much out of their bodies as they can. Often the staff join in the warming-up. It's good for them too, and it makes sense in another way – it helps them to know what their patients are experiencing. In fact, students of all disciplines will sometimes follow particular patients throughout the day, observing what happens in detail, and finding out from personal experience how they are respond-ing to their programme.

'After this patients use the gyms for an individual range of exercises and activities, with two aims: to improve the function, and to restore confidence. We've got not only the standard gym equipment, but specially designed pieces – in-cluding off-beat ones like the back of a bus (made with the co-operation of London Transport in our occupational therapy workshop), and a vaulting horse with a saddle provided by the Horse Betting Levy Board! The bus features in a popular routine. The patients are divided into two groups, one on and one off the bus. On the word "go!" those on try to get off and those off try to get on. You never saw such wielding of crutches and tripping with sticks! An excellent introduction to London Transport. As for the spirited little animal with the saddle, that's for the use of injured jockeys. We get quite a number sent by the HBLB. They're unlikely to be offered rides again until they can prove their fitness by sitting on that saddle with their stirrups shortened in that curious racing jockey crouch, and stay bouncing there as part of their final circuit. Quite a test for someone who's had a major leg injury.'

All the remedial gymnastics are under the supervision of Joan Whycherley and her staff.

Joan Whycherley worked during the war in Leicester as a GEC instrument maker. She then became a surgical corsetiere for a large department store, making, among other things, 'artificial bosoms'; she stayed there as head of department for twelve years. She had always been a gymnast, and in 1958 was selected for training for the 1960 Olympics. However, she was interested in an advertisement wanting people to train as remedial gymnasts; applied, was accepted, did an intensive 9-month course at Pinderfields General Hospital (the College of Remedial Gymnasts and Recreational Therapy, the only one at the time), qualified, came directly to the CMRC and has been there ever since.

'Remedial gymnasts were first trained during the war: initially PT instructors selected from the services to help in the recovery of injured servicemen. At first all remedial gymnasts were male, but gradually women were brought in – all from the forces. I believe I was one of the first female civilians – if not *the* first – to become a remedial gymnast. The group I was in had all been in the forces except me; there was one other woman, an officer from the WAAF.

'Now there is a full three-year course. Remedial gymnasts are trained to apply movement, re-education and recreational activity to the treatment of adults and children recovering from injury or illness, or whose physical or mental health is diminished. They also learn how to assess dosage of exercise, monitor progress, and how to relate treatment to functional activity.

'Group activity is used wherever possible: not because of the economy of the method, but because – properly applied – it extracts from each patient the most active, participatory response. The remedial gymnast has to rely on voice, manner, demonstration and leadership in order to obtain the desired response from every individual in the group.

'This isn't easy, and calls for particuar talents and character traits which a training course may develop but cannot create. Selection methods have to take account of this.

'Short-listed candidates are required to spend a full day at one of the colleges of remedial gymnastics, demonstrating to the assessors' satisfaction their ability to move well, speak well, organise and lead physical activity. The three-year training which follows is calculated to build on and develop these characteristics, and to produce therapists who can make a unique contribution to the treatment and rehabilitation of the disabled.'

HYDROTHERAPY AND OCCUPATIONAL THERAPY

Wenona Keane. 'Every day there are hydrotherapy sessions for patients in our new pool. It was part of the improvements made possible with a grant from the Hayward Foundation. The temperature of the water and the outside is kept at 90°F. In the morning the physiotherapists are in charge and treat patients on an individual basis; in the afternoon, the remedial gymnasts take in selected groups.

'After the warming-up sessions, patients separate to follow their individual programmes. Some go for occupational therapy. This isn't the old-fashioned image of making wobbly baskets to cheer themselves up. Occupational therapy is specific. Its aim is to encourage people to do things and make things in such a way that specific muscles are made to work. Of course we hope that one result is that people are pleased with the end-products, but that isn't the main point.'

Pam Court qualified at Dorset House, Oxford. She worked at Hexham Spinal Injuries Unit from 1976; after her marriage moved to the St Pancras Strokes Unit, and came to CMRC in 1978.

'It's important that we OT's *explain* to patients that occupational therapy is not a diversion. I believe its usefulness is being increasingly understood, especially as the emphasis today is on getting patients out of hospital and back home. A lot of OT's are now making home visits.

'We have three different kinds of occupational therapy here: the Activities of Daily Living training unit, light workshops, and heavy workshops.

'In the ADL training unit we help patients to tackle everyday practical problems. We give them practise in dressing themselves, shopping, cooking in a kitchen. We try to be very practical. The kitchen we have in one corner of the workroom is an ordinary kitchen, the sort you might find in any house. It's not specially designed, it hasn't got special equipment. It's got surfaces at different levels, overhead cupboards, doors that are tiresome to open, the ordinary clutter of things lying around. It's not realistic to let them cook in the sort of glossy kitchen most of them will never have when they get back home.

'Next they progress to the light workshops. Here we assess

their problems and adapt games and various creative activities to help solve them. With stroke patients in particular we aim to reduce spasticity, at the same time knowing that we may eventually have to decide to change the dominance; teaching the patient, for example, to write with the left hand rather than continue to try to re-educate the right. We're better placed than a hospital to make this decision. We see the patients at a later stage and observe them over a longer period.

'Games like pik-a-stik and dominoes train the muscles of the hand; so do skilled jobs and crafts like wiring electrical circuits or weaving seagrass. Each individual movement which is required exercises a different group of muscles.

'Because all the staff work closely together, we can back up each other's programmes. Through Joan Ellams we follow the progress patients are making with their speech, so that we can reinforce it by using pictures and flash-cards which tie in with the current sessions.

'Last of all are the heavy workshops. Not all patients are able to use these. Through our redesigned equipment they're useful for strengthening muscles, but they're also particularly valuable for those returning to jobs involving operating machinery. We use them to assess their tolerance to noise, and the sight of fast-moving machinery. Our various lathes and so on have treadles redesigned to exercise particular muscles while at the same time turning or cutting or whatever. Another important function of occupational therapy is the assessing of patients' capabilities in relation to their return to work.

'Our patients are generally very proud to take home what they make here. Anything they're not quite happy with finds a home at one of our fund-raising sales!'

PHYSIOTHERAPY

Evelyn Woolf, Head of the Physiotherapy Department, trained at West Middlesex Hospital, worked at Kingston General Hospital, and came to CMRC in 1972. She became Superintendent in 1974,

Judith McLain trained at the Middlesex (where she remembers Diana being used as a guinea-pig when students were being taught mat-work), and stayed on for two years before joining the CMRC in 1979.

'The patients attend the physiotherapy department for individual treatment. Most have at least one session daily, but this is often reduced as they improve. The treatment is very similar to that found in most physiotherapy departments; the only difference is the intensity of the treatment and the fact that we encourage active rather than passive responses.

'We aim to retrain and strengthen individual muscles, increase the mobility of specific joints, and generally improve the patients' function. All the means we use are to further this aim.

'We give assisted and resisted exercises, both by the physiotherapists alone and with the use of equipment such as springs, weights and wobble boards. All patients are also taught exercises that they can perform alone.

'We also give some electrical treatment, including ultrasonics – which promotes healing of injured tissues – and various heat treatments. We use cold therapy in the form of ice packs or baths a great deal, to relieve pain, to relax and to enable stretching of tight limbs such as found with stroke patients.

'Stroke patients also do plenty of mat-work – rolling, bridging, weight transferring, gait-training; we concentrate on trying to improve their awareness of the paralysed side, making them feel a whole person again and thus able to function more easily.'

REFERRALS

Wenona Keane. 'While all patients share in the remedial

gymnastics, physiotherapy etc., only a proportion – 10 per cent – need speech therapy. For them intensive therapy is available, both individually and in groups, with Joan Ellams*. Daily therapy such as this is available only in a handful of centres throughout the country.

'We get patients of every age and from every background.

'We try to achieve a balance of approximately 60 per cent short-term (mainly orthopaedic patients) to 40 per cent medical (which includes the stroke patients). Patients may come as a result of illnesses, such as multiple sclerosis, or accidents, either at work or through sport or on the road. In the younger groups we get a large number of young men injured on motor cycles: one particular week all the admissions on both Monday and Tuesday were motor cyclists. We also get a disproportionate number of males: 80 per cent to 20 per cent females. This is far more marked among people in their teens and early twenties, partly because up till now more males have had dangerous jobs – in the docks, the building trades, demolition, mining – and more dangerous hobbies.

'Half of our patients go back to their old jobs. Of the others, approximately 18 per cent will never work again. The remainder need reassessment to be able to switch to different work. They may need to be referred to the Disablement Resettlement Officer at their local Jobcentre to help them with this.'

WHAT REHABILITATION CAN ACHIEVE
Dr JGS is Medical Director of Rehabilitation at the CMRC. He is also Director of the Department of Rheumatology and Rehabilitation at University College Hospital, Chairman of the North-Eastern Region Health Authority's Advisory Sub-Committee on Rehabilitation and Rheumatology, the British member of Rehabilitation International, and Adviser on the

* See pages 59, 86

Rehabilitation Department of Social Affairs for the EEC. 'He eats, drinks and breathes rehabilitation.'

'There's nothing magic in the treatment people get here. The equipment we have is no different from what you'd find in most hospitals – indeed, in many cases theirs would be better. Our staff have had the same training. They use the same techniques. The only difference is the concentration of attention which is available here. Our patients get more treatment in one day than in one week in a good hospital.

'On the whole, most of our patients are of working age, and our aim is, if possible, to get them back to work again. You have to start the rehabilitation early enough. Otherwise, a disabled and unemployed person after a period of time becomes a disabled and unemployable person. If they're left too long, they don't want to work. They may not like the life they're leading, but they feel threatened by the mere thought of work. While, if we get them soon enough, and provided they're well enough to live at home and come here daily, something can be done for almost everyone.

'Medical opinion too often confines itself to observant neglect of the disabled – through ignorance of what's available, or total lack of facilities. We understand here that patients must *work* to get better, not *wait* to get better.

'We can't make people come here, nor compel them to attend regularly once they do. Yet our percentage attendance is virtually 100 per cent. The fact is that people *enjoy* themselves here. This seems to be a constant surprise to doctors and medical students who come and see us. I say to them "Would you rather they were miserable? Of course they enjoy getting better and feeling themselves getting better. Wouldn't you?" But they're still astonished at the atmosphere here.

'We owe an enormous amount to our staff and their enthusiasm. They get something here too. They get job satisfaction. Our patients are individuals, not just disabilities. None of your "tib and fib in bed 3". Our staff can watch people improve. When we extended two years ago I refused to take in any more patients. We have as many as we can manage, so that staff and patients all know each other. That's why, unlike even the best hospitals with excellent reputations, we seldom have any difficulty in getting staff – even domestic staff. We have waiting lists of people wanting to come.

'We make economic sense too. The total cost *per day* per patient is less than one isolated out-patient attendance at a teaching hospital. And that includes meals – *and* the constant intravenous drip of tea without which no one in the country seems able to survive. Looked at in the loss of work-time, too, rehabilitation pays off. It's the *total* time off work which counts. The average time off work for a patient with a broken leg is nine months. Rehabilitation could often cut this down and put the patient back in circulation much earlier: better for him, better for society.

'We had a striking demonstration of what therapy can do. Originally we gave hemiplegics speech therapy three times a week: 21 per cent went back to paid employment. We stepped the therapy up to three times a day five times a week: and 43 per cent went back to paid employment. Double the number of people had their life prospects improved, yet the only change was the increase in speech therapy.

'For all patients with speech disabilities early and intensive therapy is vital. We sometimes get notes from a hospital which state that "X had speech therapy and did not benefit." Then when we look further we find that the patient had an hour's therapy once a week. Of course there was no benefit, or no noticeable benefit. Any improvement at that level would be so slight as to be unmeasurable. What's upsetting is that someone reading those notes without our experience may conclude that further speech therapy is pointless, and the patient will simply not be adequately treated.

'There is far too little appreciation in the medical profession of what rehabilitation can do. In only three of the great London teaching hospitals is there any instruction on the benefits of occupational therapy, physiotherapy and speech therapy. In all of the others it is possible for doctors to qualify knowing nothing whatever about these. There is colossal medical ignorance.

'We are very conscious that as a result we are not treating the patients who need us. We merely treat those who are referred to us. The rest will not get the treatment they need. As it is, we know that in many cases the impetus for referrals comes from occupational therapists or even neighbours; the direct referral comes from a GP or through the hospital, of course, but that's only the end-result – the initial inspiration was elsewhere.

'We need more rehabilitation centres like ours: several small ones rather than one large central one. Travel time and the expense of transport otherwise create insuperable barriers. Ideally, there should also be a small number of beds available for those who live too far from any centre. We ourselves could do with say six hostel beds here.

'There is increasing interest in rehabilitation, as evidenced by the frequent borrowings of our recent film, *Return to Life*. On our open days we have people visiting here not only from all over the country but from all over the world. In 1978 we had 984 visitors from fourteen countries; in 1979 visitors from nineteen countries.

'Rehabilitation not only improves the life of the individual, but it is cost-effective. Our hope is that its importance is becoming increasingly appreciated.'

8 'No more sitting at home'

Such was to be the background of Diana's life for the next eleven busy and fruitful months, ferried to and from the Centre by ambulance each weekday morning and evening. Many of those who helped Diana are still there today, and combine to give a picture of her at that time when, as she herself recalls with gratitude, there was 'no more sitting at home.'

Dr JGS. 'Diana's success demonstrates two vital factors: the importance of the motivation and the influence of the family.

'Diana was absolutely determined to succeed. She made the most of her possibilities, and constantly drove herself on. In rehabilitation, the motivation behind the patient is perhaps what matters most of all – more than the extent of the initial disability. It's interesting that research shows that self-employed people recover much more quickly than the employed. Of course, the relationship isn't as simple as it looks – the self-employed tend to be more determined, more individualistic by their nature, and in most cases they've got more interesting jobs to go back to – but it does show that what counts is the individual determination to improve. It's the fighting spirit; and that's what Diana's got.

'Almost as important – in fact, in a negative way it can turn out to be equally important – is the kind of help and reaction the patient gets from his or her family. It's the total situation which counts; again, far more important than the actual disability. The husband or wife or other relative can support the individual's struggle for achievement; or they can destroy it.

'Most often they do this by being over-kind, over-protective. We aim here to teach each individual to be as independent as possible. It's destructive for them to go back home and find that something they've worked at for hours over many days to achieve is done for them in a few seconds by a "helpful" relative. It destroys their self-confidence and their will to work at their progress.

'I know it's hard for relatives to watch a wife or husband or whatever struggling to do a simple thing like walking to fetch a newspaper or pour a cup of tea, and it's perfectly natural to want to do it for them, but they must understand that it's the opposite of helpful. Diana got the right sort of back-up from those around her, and especially – and over a long period – from her mother.

'Right next to the family I should include friends. They can have a very important part to play. At the same time, it's fair to point out that not everyone – friend or relative – can cope with the results of an illness like this. Some will stick, and others won't. I feel myself that those who don't perhaps shouldn't blame themselves too much. We all have different capacities.

'Over-helpfulness can also hinder speech recovery. Often relatives and friends understand what a patient means when there's very little verbal communication at all. It's the same in any ordinary family: people understand each other with very few words when an outsider wouldn't. But relatives can help by not relying on the odd words and a few gestures, but by encouraging the husband or wife to put his or her meanings into words. Otherwise, there's no progress towards improved communication with others *outside* the family. Helping the individual towards speech, however limited, breaks down their isolation.

'It does take time. It can be exhausting on both sides. And progress can be dishearteningly slow. But it's the only way.

'The example of another of our patients, Douglas Ritchie*, demonstrates the need (and the reward) of persistence and continuity. He began to write his diary of a stroke as part of his speech therapy, with no thought of publication. His therapist helped him to work on a sentence a day, over and over again, until the final version was recorded. Clearly, this meant an immense amount of dedication and effort.

'Relatives can help not only by encouraging speech, and by understanding how slow progress can be, but in other more subtle ways which may be obvious if you think about it, but perhaps aren't if you don't. Involve the person concerned in what's going on. Leave them to hand round the sandwiches or pour out the drink. Bring them into the conversation. When their speech is still very limited, ask questions which need only short answers, or even just yes or no. It's easy to talk round someone, but it doesn't take that much more thought to include them, and it makes a lot of difference. With many people, it's best to keep away from abstract ideas, and to rephrase thoughts into concrete terms.

SPEECH THERAPY AND THE QUALITY OF LIFE

'Yes, I agree with Diana that of course we need more speech therapists, but we're unlikely to ever get enough. I'm a member of the executive of the Chest Heart and Stroke Association and on their Stroke Committee, and the kind of clubs the Association helps to organise are always glad to have the advice of speech therapists. But when it's unavailable, and in between times, volunteer help means there's something useful going on. At the very least, it improves communication possibilities and the chances of those who participate.

* See Appendix 1

'I believe speech therapists now mainly go along with this. When Valerie Eaton Griffiths first wrote her book, *A Stroke in the Family*, with her account of how friends helped Patricia Neal with her speech difficulties, she got an enormous amount of opposition from speech therapists who felt that she was daring to suggest that professional help was replaceable by amateurs. She's always very particular now to stress that voluntary helpers are not quasi-therapists, but can nonetheless contribute in their own way.

'Diana's often critical about the sceptical attitude of various medical authorities to speech therapy. I can understand her feelings. There are doctors and consultants who don't give therapy the support they should. They question the time and effort involved in producing what they see as often only a very small improvement. Joan Ellams would say that this is not the point. Speech therapy, even though it may not – indeed probably won't – bring back the kind of speech that was there before, makes better communication possible, and immeasurably improves the quality of life.

'There's often too much emphasis on a quantitative result in medicine. For example, I'm concerned in encouraging riding for the disabled. Now, since we don't use horses for getting around any more, it doesn't make the individual more mobile. It can strengthen their legs so they can walk better. But above all the sheer happiness and the sense of well-being that they can get from riding can't be measured.

'I remember some shots in a film we made on this riding – marvellous camerawork. You see a small boy throw himself from his wheel chair and crawl and pull himself through the grass. Then you see him struggle to drag himself up a five-barred gate. Then you watch him pull and heave himself into the saddle, and sit upright. And you see all this from the boy's viewpoint. First of all long grass at his eye-level. Then the bars of the gate one by one. And finally from his head right up there on the horse and looking around and below him at what he saw. You can imagine what his face was like. It was one enormous beam.

'That's the kind of thing we try to promote here. We try to encourage every individual in every way so that they can make the most of the possibilities of their life.

'And of course Diana has gone on to do just that.

'I feel though that I ought to point out two things which are inter-connected. Diana is an exceptional person who has made an exceptional recovery; it would be wrong to raise false hopes in the relatives of stroke patients and lead them to *expect* that such an achievement is always or even frequently attainable. Yet, at the same time, most people – given motivation and the right help – can make astonishing progress. Even when considerable impairment remains, as is most often the case, a useful and fruitful life can still be led.

'I hope Diana won't mind my saying that although her comprehension is very good, and has improved tremendously since she first came here, it is to some degree imperfect. Her speech too, although it is very adequate, is not what it was. She has to rely on a pattern of phrases to get her meaning across, and inevitably the subtleties that she must want to convey are lost. Nonetheless, in spite of these impairments, she has managed to do so much. She's a good organiser and she knows how to pick people. She has made her talents work for her.

'Before her stroke, she was obviously a highly intelligent and successful person heading for the top. But now, she's doing something that no one else but someone with her background and capacities could possibly do. She has the understanding from her personal experience of what a stroke is and can do to a person, the temperament and background to make her determined to make use of what has happened to her for the general good, the capacity to know what to do, and the determination to go ahead and do it.'

'BOTH SIDES OF THE FENCE'

Reg Black. Two accidents, followed by a mistaken double anti-tetanus injection, ended his twenty-six years in the London and Essex Fire Services and brought him to the CMRC with partial paralysis of both arms. After his recovery he began working there, at first as a transport officer, and then in various other capacities. He is now Administration Officer.

'My view of what goes on here must be a bit different from anyone else's, because I see things from both sides of the fence, you might say. I started here as a patient, like Diana, though not as badly disabled as she was, and then, after I was discharged, I came here to work.

'I think Diana would probably agree with me that what made the most tremendous difference right from the word go was the wonderful welcome I got. When they came to me whilst I was attending hospital as an out-patient, they said they couldn't do anything more for me and told me about this place, where I could attend every single week-day. They told me, "If they can't help you no one can," and I thought to myself, who've they got there? God? I had no idea what to expect, and I was really apprehensive.

'But the moment I arrived, I got the most beaming smile of greeting you can imagine. It made all the difference to me. I felt wanted. I felt I was an individual. All that first morning, as I was taken round from place to place, everywhere I went I was introduced, and everybody behaved the same way, doctors, sisters, the other people. Everyone was so friendly.

'And everyone *explained* things to me, so I knew what was going on. When the doctor and the nurses went down to the other end of the room and started talking to each other, the sister said to me, "Don't worry, there's nothing wrong, all they're doing is discussing the best programme for you. We won't keep anything from you. Any time you want to know anything, just ask."

'I felt elated.

'Mind you, I didn't feel so elated next day when the treatment started! It's hard work. It's very hard work. It's a combination of kindness and pressure, worked out for the individual. You're helped, not forced. The programme's tailored for you. That's why people like Diana and me could make such progress here. The hospitals simply can't cope in the same way. They haven't the time or the staff to give the intensive care that's needed. I used to have more treatment in one morning than in one week attending hospital. And Diana was worse than I was when she arrived. To be so badly handicapped in speech – it's very frustrating. But she was helped to persevere. That's the real secret here.

'The staff look at every patient individually all the time. It's all psychological. Nothing's allowed to stay stagnant. Once a week, the whole staff meets through a Tuesday lunchtime, and they discuss every single patient's progress. So that every single patient gets moved along as soon as they're ready. They start on the ground floor and work up, so to speak.

'The whole staff is dedicated to helping. Many stay for years. Even the domestic staff, they're all part of the team. It's very rewarding. When you see someone arrive in a wheel-chair, and you watch them walk out, you feel ten foot tall.

'In my opinion we need far more day centres like this. They'd help to take some of the pressure off the hospitals, and people would be able to pick up the threads of their lives much more quickly. In particular, with stroke patients like Diana, we could do more if they were referred to us as early as possible.

'Someone like Diana shows what can be done. It's a shame

to think there must be people all over the place who could profit from the same sort of help, but who just aren't going to get it.'

A PHYSICAL CHALLENGE

Wenona Keane. 'I was Head of the OT Department when Diana first came. Two of us went with her on the original home visit to her own flat. We got on well – partly because she discovered I was about one-eighth Irish! I saw to part of her treatment, which was carried out on a day-to-day basis by other OT's; and I had many chats with her. She had tremendous problems, but she was fighting hard.

'Her ADL (Activities of Daily Living) file has a detailed report of what she had achieved after the first two months: including dressing, washing, bed-making, cleaning, opening bottles and screw-top jars. She could cut her nails using clippers for her right hand and a file attached to a block for her left. She had difficulty with public transport: she was so slow that if the conductor failed to notice her getting on a bus it could be dangerous. She couldn't strike matches, but said it didn't matter as she didn't use them. She could only carry small parcels. She couldn't put up an ironing board, but said she didn't iron much anyway and could manage on a table. Most of the housework was done by the cleaner. As for cooking: "She has made biscuits, meringues and three lunches. Can manage to peel potatoes but doesn't eat them at home."

'Her main problem with independent living was bathing independence. At that time she needed "minimal help" from her mother. "No bath aid except non-skid mat."

'Various small aids were suggested: a modified washing-up rack, a hot-water bottle holder, a wall tin opener, and so on. Diana contributed to the cost, and by the time she was discharged her flat had been equipped to help her lead an independent life. On a physical level, she achieved a very considerable success.'

Joan Whycherley. 'I always remember Diana from the moment she arrived. She hadn't much movement. She could hardly speak. I remember she used to say "My dear!" and "But but but," and "Marvellous!" And what was that when she disapproved? That's right – "NO-O-O!" Very long drawn-out and emphatic.

'But she impressed me very early on with her quiet determination to succeed. Nothing was too much trouble for her. She never grumbled. Whatever it was she'd always have a go, to show it could be done.

'Part of Diana's programme was to join in a group we call Early Activities. The first aim in this group is to improve morale. To this end, patients are encouraged to see their disabilities in perspective. This is only possible in a group situation with other patients with other disabilities. By working in a group like this, it's possible for the patient to see somebody worse off than – or at least as badly off as him or herself. Most people come to feel that they can cope better with their own disabilities than they could with someone else's. Better the devil you know . . .

'Other aims of this group include strengthening muscles and making patients more mobile; there are also various activities to improve co-ordination and speed. Most important of all, though, is the underlying aim: to help patients to function as nearly normally as possible, and thus enable them to achieve independence.

'We start at the basics and go on from there. The very first step is for them to get down on the floor and up again. Then we get them to walk across the gym. They'll start by clinging to the wall bars. They're frightened of empty space. When they can do that, we take them into the street. They learn to walk on uneven pavements, getting used to the noise and hubbub of people and passing traffic, preparing themselves for going out on real buses. Inside, they walk up and down stairs. Diana would be off up to the top, always ready to be in the lead. Not show off, but to encourage.

'She always accepted a challenge. There's one exercise we do, I put two benches at an angle leading up and down to a vaulting box. It takes a lot of nerve, when one leg is paralysed and you've not much sense of balance, to walk up those benches. Diana wouldn't hesitate. She'd be up there in a moment. Just by what she did she gave courage to others.

'It's not an easy thing to get, confidence, and even with someone like Diana it doesn't take a lot to destroy it. There was one thing that made me very angry – I don't know whether Diana remembers. When she'd been coming to us for some while, her mother needed a holiday and, to give her a break, Diana went into hospital for a month. It was arranged that to make things easier all round she would continue her treatment there.

'Now before she went into hospital she was already sufficiently independent to go to the shops at the end of the road – we send a therapist as well, but at a little distance, to keep an eye open and see nothing happens – to go out and buy simple things for herself. Well, when she came back from the hospital all that independence had vanished. A thoughtless remark by a therapist had shattered her confidence, saying her "walking pattern was appalling," and that "Camden should get their priorities right."

'It seems to me important to temper one's enthusiasm with a sense of realism. There comes a time with many patients when you have to stop being super-scientific and go for confidence and function at any price. Bearing in mind that there is a one in six chance of a further stroke within a year, most patients would probably prefer to spend their time with their families rather than practise a perfect gait pattern as a long-term patient in a long-term unit.

'It took weeks for Diana to regain her confidence. Sometimes I would give her individual therapy. One day, I remember, I gave her a balancing exercise to perform. I put a bench on a thick rubber mat – that makes it wobbly.

Then I told Diana to stand on the bench, hold on to the wall-bars, and deliberately wobble the bench. Then she had to leave go of the bars, stand there and wobble it again. Then I told her to hold on to the bars, and stand only on her good foot. So she tried that. I told her that next session she'd be standing only on her weak foot. She just made a face, stood there, lifted up her good foot, and stood there wobbling away on her weak one! That was the old Diana spirit returning, and I knew we were winning.'

'SEVERE EXPRESSIVE DYSPHASIA'

For Diana, the most important of all the benefits of the CMRC was the intensive speech therapy she received there.

Some people think leg matters. For me, no. Speech is first.

Joan Ellams. 'Diana's initial report in January 1969 describes her as "a pleasant, cheerful lady with severe expressive dysphasia."

'It's important to remember that "dysphasia*" isn't the same for everyone, with identical causes and effects and treatment. Diana initially had *dyspraxia*: she would be unable to get her mouth to form the word even though she knew what it was and even though there was no physical reason – in the movements of her mouth, tongue and so on – why she couldn't. (Some stroke patients suffer from *dysarthria*: the motor muscles of the mouth are affected so that they're unable to speak but may be able to write. Diana doesn't suffer from this.) Diana still has dyspraxia on occasion, but very much less than she did.

'She also had a lot of *verbal paraphasia*. This means that the individual uses the wrong word, but it's one which in *idea* has some connection with the right one. Diana might say "butter" instead of "cheese" or "June" instead

* See also page 155

of "August." She also had something called *literal para-phasia*, which involves the transfer of sounds from one part of the word to another. For example, she might say "puc" for "cup."

'My notes also indicate that she had "auditory percep-tive difficulty." This means that although she had no hearing difficulties she would confuse similar sounds – like Ps and Bs and Ts and Ds. She could hear and distinguish between the sounds. If I showed her pictures of "tart" and "dart", she would point to the picture corresponding to what I said, but be unable to pick the right sound when she attempted to speak the word.

'On the other hand, she had almost no *perseveration*, which can affect many dysphasics. This means that they persist in using one word for a number of objects; they correctly recall the word "table" for "table", but go on using it to mean "dress" or "chair" as well.

'Dysphasia affects *all* aspects of language. It's very rare for a dysphasic to be able to write but not speak, while someone suffering from dysarthria can. Without speech, dysphasics have only very limited possibilities of com-munication.

The actual therapy programme varies with each indivi-dual, though of course there are some elements in com-mon. With Diana, I started by working on the compre-hension of spoken language. I would get her to respond to simple orders like "Open the book," "Pick up the box." Then I would get her to match objects on the table to words. "Show me the pencil," "Show me the dominoes," and so on. Then we went on to simple questions that she could answer with one word.

'We also worked on written words. I would read aloud a short paragraph in very simple English and show it to Diana. I would underline the key words, or outline them in a different colour, and then ask her questions. To begin with, she would point to the answers; later she would try to say the words. For writing, we would work on associating letter shapes with sounds. She found this difficult, and still does.

'Later still, we worked on expressive language. It's not re-learning. It's practising recall. We use various devices to prompt the brain – like finding words through sentences. I would say, "The boy is riding on his . . ." and Diana would add "bicycle." Or I might give her a sentence which could have several possible answers. " The boy was eating a . . ." leaving Diana to pick the word she wanted. Often it would help her if I prompted her with the initial syllable, or even an initial letter.

'In April 1969 she did the same Eisonson test she had previously done in June 1968. In ten months she had made considerable progress. Her reading was little better, so was her writing, but although she still had some receptive diffi- culties both her comprehension and her speech had im- proved. She spoke very slowly, and one word would stand for a complex idea. "Chair" might mean "sit down" or "The chair is broken" or "I want the chair recovered."

'Diana continued to make progress all the time she was here – and of course later. She's never stopped. But none of it was easy for her. She was very emotional when she first came – this is part of the effects of the stroke. She would burst into tears of frustration, but she usually man- aged to get a hold of herself and become common-sensical again.

'From the point of view of speech and language Diana is very typical of the development of an average stroke patient; but from the point of view of her personality she isn't at all. She has initiative, courage and determination. These were all characteristics that she had before, and she's brought them through the stroke with her. She is active, not passive. She has qualities of leadership.

'Professionally, Diana has been a great help to me. She's very bossy! The moment she heard about a new

MSc course in 1970, she said I had to do it. She kept on about it, organising me, until in the end I did it to shut her up. I worked in my own time for two years. I got a half-day release from here to work at Guy's, and I had lectures two evenings a week. I wrote a paper which looked into the relationship between cognitive ability and dysphasia. It was hard work, but I enjoyed it, and I almost certainly wouldn't have done it if Diana hadn't nagged me into it.

'Others can recover as well or better than she has, but they won't have the same determination to communicate. They won't do as much with what they recapture. Her speech when she left here was still very little. It's what she's done with it that matters.

'The more I see of patients, the more I feel that what influences what they do with their lives after their strokes is what they made of their lives before.

'Some may recover well enough to return to their jobs, but others may have to return to family life and rely on their own hobbies and interests. Those with a good marriage and a good family life can and do cope.

'Often there's no reason why they can't do what they did and what they want to do, but at a different level. One of my patients was a solicitor in his forties. He made a fair recovery, but not enough for him to go back to the law. He'd always been interested in painting and paintings, and he opened an art gallery. He was very keen on sailing – in fact he was an Olympic racer; he sold his boat and bought another which was easier to manage. He still goes sailing, but with his family, and on a different scale.

'I've another patient who was an engineer but made a not very good recovery. He always liked gardening, and now with his wife's help they have a greenhouse and do intensive all-year-round gardening.

'But of course this sort of thing isn't open to everyone. It can be very hard for those who have always had few interests outside work. It means looking forward to a life of retirement, but prematurely, and often in poor health. It can be an uphill task, not only for the patient but for all their family. It can be a hard cross to bear. But without wanting to sound falsely optimistic, I would like to say that there are more possibilities and a better life than might seem possible.'

TIME TO GO

I'm happy! Then, same as the Wolfson, they tell me it's time to go. Not enough notice. People like me, you must give them time to adjust. I thought I would be there for weeks, months, years! Suddenly, I was at home again.

Joan Ellams. 'She was very upset when the time came for her to leave the Centre. We had tears for several weeks. I was tempted to go on sick leave at the time! If Diana says she had short notice, it's because she doesn't want to remember. It's common with many of our patients. They're happy here. Their days are full. They make friends. They have a purpose in life. Many of them don't want to go back to their homes. They block off the thought that one day they'll have to.

'It's not easy for us. We're dealing with adults. We're trying to enable them to be as independent as possible, to take charge of their own lives. We don't want to destroy what we're doing by constantly referring over their heads to relatives.

'Diana was told a long time in advance when she would be due to leave, but she dogmatically wouldn't tell anyone. She probably really accepted it only two or three days before.

'But we didn't just turf her out with no forethought. We made arrangements for her to have group therapy – at the City Lit, the Middlesex and the College of Speech Sciences – and to go on having treatment from me; and for her to come back here for short refresher courses. But there is a time when even the longest-stay patients – and Diana was one, she was here for nearly twelve months – have to leave and go back to their own lives.

'It's never easy.'

9   Biding time

Diana devoted the next couple of years to consolidating and building upon the progress she had already made.

At one time she had intended to return to her own flat and live apart from her mother, but in the event she never did.

Joan Ellams. 'Her mother was understandably anxious about what might happen if Diana was entirely on her own, and I think that possibly, in spite of what she said, Diana was herself apprehensive too.'

So, from this time on, while Diana occasionally used her old flat to entertain friends or for her speech therapy, she continued to camp out, as it were, in her mother's flat: a mutually supportive arrangement.

The recovery of speech, and thus the importance of speech therapy, continued to be of prime importance. She carried on with her two (private) hourly sessions with Joan Ellams. Once a week she walked to the National Hospitals College of Speech Sciences for speech therapy with Michael Jackson. Twice a week she went to the Middlesex Hospital – a walk taking forty-five minutes there and forty-five back – for thirty minutes individual speech therapy and an hour's occupational therapy.

Catherine Taylor trained at St George's Hospital; and after working in various hospitals and private clinics left to work in America and Canada. She then joined the Middlesex Hospital to work first as ward sister, then night sister, and eventually in the Out-Patients Department. She transferred in 1974 to Nursing Administration.

'I met Diana for the first time in an informal way back in the 1970s. I used to see her in Out-Patients when she was waiting for her speech therapy. She had had her stroke only a short time before, and she had very little speech. I was most impressed. She was very brave. She *always* spoke to us, making huge efforts to communicate.'

Twice a week she was taken by car (paid for by Westminster City Council) to the City Literary Institute for two hours of group speech therapy with Peggy Dalton.

Peggy Dalton graduated in English from Oxford and then acted (as Peggy Butt) for ten years. Becoming increasingly interested in speech and language, she trained as a speech therapist – on a grant – at the then Oldrey-Fleming School of Speech Therapy, now merged with the National Hospitals College of Speech Sciences. She then worked for two years at two part-time jobs: at the University College Hospital and at a school for physically handicapped children. She left to divide her time between the Middlesex Hospital and the City Literary Institute. She now teaches and is a therapist at the School for the Study of Disorders of Human Communication at Blackfriars.

'Diana was an early member of one of our first groups at the City Lit. I had about eight members at each session, all stroke patients except for one with Parkinson's disease, and all referrals from other therapists at various hospitals. At first the groups were held once a week, then twice, then three times, then finally every day. Each session lasted two hours. Most people came from two to three times a week.

'Just by chance this happened to be a particularly advanced group, which helped Diana find the kind of stimulus she needed. The general level of comprehension was good, so we were able to concentrate on high-level work. Anyone with severe difficulties in comprehension should only work in groups of people with similar problems, or the individuals concerned risk becoming very frustrated.

'Diana's comprehension at that time was good, but her speech was very limited. She still had only a few simple words. Mostly she used them appropriately, and provided the listener knew what the context was she would manage to get her message across.

'In the group my aim was to stimulate and improve their ability to communicate. I wasn't interested primarily in accuracy. I wanted to improve their confidence in their own abilities, and help them to get their thoughts and emotions across.

'I used various treatments, working first on communication and the spoken language. We did different kinds of speech exercises, using them always in a flexible way. I might choose a theme. For example, I'd put up a large map of London with the different monuments marked, and ask members of a group to comment on what this evoked. You might get reminiscences, or details of tube travel, or descriptions of famous places, or suggestions for walks. Some might speak a little, some more. They'd fill in for each other, or set up reactions from each other. Then I might have pictures of famous people, and go on from there. It's useful to have controversial figures. People get het up and want to argue. Or I might play different kinds of music and see what that evoked.

'We'd do a certain amount of role playing, asking members of the group to imagine themselves in different situations and having to express what they would want to say.

'I'd encourage them to try some reading. Writing they

could tackle or not as they pleased. It's more important for some individuals than others; they can make their own decisions about how to spend their time.

'Diana continued to improve. She was always determined to *work* at getting better. You could see how single-minded she was. During our groups she wasn't satisfied just to concentrate on speech, she would work at the physical side at the same time. She'd sit there raising her arms over her head, doing her exercises, manipulating her hands. She'd walk around the room to exercise her legs, and so on. Diana's a tremendous fighter. She wears her speech therapists out! She has great will-power, and a ferocity and self-conviction which is absolutely necessary for what she has accomplished.'

Joan Ellams. 'In 1972 she was assessed using the *Minnesota test for the differential diagnosis of dysphasia.* Her speech and language were very much improved since the last test in 1970. She still had some difficulty in comprehension, mainly when she had to deal with particularly long or complex matters. Even so, it was largely a question of concentrating.

'When you're dysphasic, you *must* concentrate. You can't half listen to things, as we all tend to do. You really have to listen, full stop. She would miss details sometimes. She tended to be a bad listener; she probably always was. People are either listeners or talkers, and Diana's a great talker.'

Later, looking back, Diana in her prize-winning essay through the help of Joan Ellams summed up her progress at this point.

I noticed that I was having much less difficulty in understanding what was being said to me. I was now even able to understand my accountant when discussing my somewhat complicated financial position. . . . I could cope with the headlines in the newspaper and even with short articles and with letters from friends, but anything more complicated just led to confusion and loss of interest. As for spoken language. . . . as the months went by I acquired a larger vocabulary . . . but as for writing down my thoughts and ideas I simply could not. It was proving impossible to write anything other than my name and address.

INDEPENDENCE

In personal terms too Diana continued to make progress. By now she could do virtually everything for herself.

At first Jacqueline washed my hair. My mother bathed me. Jacqueline washed my clothes in the Wolfson. Now I do everything myself. I bath myself, wash my hair, wash my clothes, everything.

Mary Law. 'Within the flat she became completely independent. She has a little washboard for her own washing. She can use the grill and prepare vegetables. She washes dishes and dries up. She even uses the carpet sweeper. She walks around a great deal in the flat. It helps to give her exercise.'

Friends called to see her. She went out visiting. She invited people in for meals.

Wenona Keane. 'After she left she went on using her flat from time to time. I remember once she invited me to supper there. I still have her letter, which she wrote herself. It was one of the best composed letters I have ever had. It went:
Dear Miss Keane,
1. Happy New Year.

2, Supper?

3. Her address, printed on a piece of paper, stuck on.

4. The date.

5. OK?

6. Diana Law.

'And I went and had an excellent supper and a very pleasant evening.'

She kept in close touch with the CMRC, returning for a check-up in January 1970, for a three-week refresher course in July 1970, and for a further three weeks in February 1971 and January 1972.

She had also started again on what were to become her regular twice-yearly visits to Osborne*: by now a much looked forward to social event.

But during all this time, beyond her own immediate concerns, Diana never forgot the pledge she had made herself in those first terrible days in hospital: to do her best to help those 'silent people' – as she was later to describe them – who could do nothing to help themselves.

Already in 1971 Diana, with her friends, was starting to break out of her own immediate circle to seek help for those more handicapped than herself.

The notes for a meeting held (with the assistance of Felicity Lane-Fox and Anne Handley-Derry) with Lady Masham in December 1971 are typical of several at this time.

Most grateful for interview and for Lady Masham getting in touch with Lord Aberdare. Anxious to hear his comments but wish to stress again that my original letter was *not* to ask for help myself but for others who cannot bring their needs to public attention. No public

* See page 129

D

money is provided to help those with speech handicaps. Are they a forgotten section of the community?

The notes go on to enquire about: the provision of buses for speech-handicapped people wishing to attend at the City Literary Institute; the possibility of sheltered accommodation for younger disabled people; employment potentials; recreational facilities; the provision of tape recorders.

With the ready help and encouragement of her friends, Diana pressed on with the pursuit of many inter-related issues affecting those handicapped people she felt society ignored.

Then, in 1972, with the help of her friend Jean Lewis, Diana sent the *Daily Telegraph* on October 4th the letter which was henceforth to encourage her to focus her energies on one specific issue: the promotion of speech clubs for the speech-handicapped.

10 'Communication always my job'

'Communication always my job' says Diana; and in 1972 she worked out what needed doing and how best to go about it.

The problem, as she saw it, had three elements.

One: She knew from her own experience that those whose speech was damaged or totally absent – whether as a result of damage to the brain or to the vocal cords – would not simply recover their speech with time. What was needed was the professional help of therapists who would instruct and encourage their patients to produce speech in a different way. Yet she had discovered that this skilled help was in many cases not available at all; and even when it was, perhaps only once or twice a week for as little as half an hour a time. This contrasted poorly indeed with her own intensive therapy at the CMRC.

Two: This neglect, this inadequate and infrequent therapy, was inevitable, as long as there were so few trained speech therapists available (at that time less than 200 working in all the hospitals in England and Wales to deal with all the speech problems faced by patients recovering from strokes, head injuries, Parkinson's disease, brain tumours and laryngectomies).

Three: (an even longer-term proposition): The situation would not be remedied until both the general public *and* the medical hierarchy (often astonishingly ignorant about the aims and achievements of speech therapy) could be educated to understand what was involved and how many people were suffering, and to vote for the expanded speech therapy training programme which was needed.

Meanwhile, help was needed for those already suffering in silence.

Diana again drew from her own experience.

Although individual speech therapy would obviously remain the ideal, Diana knew how much benefit she had received from group therapy at the CMRC, and was still receiving regularly at the City Lit. At these sessions a number of speech handicapped people could receive skilled help from one trained person.

What was needed, in the short term, was to follow this example and make these precious facilities available to more people.

Diana talked this over with her friend Jean Lewis. It was decided to start the ball rolling with a letter to the *Daily Telegraph*.

Jean Lewis worked as secretary for various MPs, the last being Basil de Ferranti. When Ferranti Ltd sold their computer department to ICL, and Basil de Ferranti went as Managing Director, Jean Lewis went with him. Here she met Diana for the first time. She later went to work for Timothy Sainsbury, and is now their Press Officer.

'I kept in touch with Diana after her stroke. I was trying to think of how we might gauge the response of people to her idea of stroke* clubs, and I felt that a letter to the *Daily Telegraph* might help us to assess how many people might in fact be affected. At that time her speech was still too limited for her to be able to frame it herself. So I drafted it. It was using the kind of expertise I had anyway in my job. I interpreted what I thought she wanted to say, and then we talked it over together. I'm sure I then made

* Later to be called 'speech clubs'

many alterations in response to her ideas. Then we sent it off.'

It appeared on October 4th under the heading of 'Stroke Clubs.'

SIR,

I wonder how many of your readers who suffer from speech disorders following brain damage, or who have relatives or friends in this situation, would be interested in joining with me in representing more widely the particular interests of this group? Official figures do not specify the number of those who have speech disabilities of this sort as opposed to those who are classified as 'deaf without speech' but I believe it to be sufficiently large to be worthy of a great deal more attention.

Four and a half years ago I had a severe stroke which left me unable to speak at all for about two years, and paralysed my right side. Although I have now to a certain extent overcome the disability of the paralysis, I still have great difficulty in speaking and am unable to write.

I have met a sad lack of awareness of the special problems confronting those who want to learn to speak again. It seems that it is only through the very devoted efforts of speech therapists, who see the importance of immediate treatment, one's own family and friends, and limited facilities in certain institutions that any progress can be made. I count myself among the lucky ones having had immeasurable help and support in my efforts to regain my speech.

I have in mind the forming of 'stroke clubs' in areas where a sufficient number of people would be willing to get together.

Diana Law

Jean Lewis wrote it for me. It was posted in Osborne. I was staying with Daphne on the way back when it was printed. I wanted to know . . . Me alone? Or others? Afterwards there were a lot, a very lot of letters! That was the start of my speech clubs. Slow beginning. Very slow! But now many clubs. We must have more.

Jean Lewis. 'After it appeared Diana got these heart-rending letters. Over 200. Each one of them a personal tragedy. I think Diana's letter encouraged them to look beyond themselves, to realise there were others in the same position.'

Mary Law. 'When Diana's letter was published she found her purpose in life. She had found her goal; and she went straight ahead.'

THE FIRST SPEECH CLUBS

The publication of her letter, and the response it brought, started Diana off on the road she has followed ever since, to promote speech clubs – and incidentally to encourage the many individuals who have written to her – throughout the world.

The first club to be founded after the letter's publication – and a subsequent report in Diana's local paper, the *Mercury* – was under the auspices of Westminster City Council; to be followed not long afterwards by another (no longer in existence) founded by Stephen Monaghan in Area 5 of Camden Borough; and then by one (now in Quintin Kynaston school) started by Diana with the help of Barbara Deason.

Barbara Deason started by working in Camden Welfare Department, helping principally the handicapped and the elderly. She trained as a social worker at Coventry before returning to Camden in 1971 to do two years' generic social work. She then became a community worker, working with local groups and organisations; and during this period first met Diana. She has since moved to Wandsworth, first as senior practitioner for the physically handicapped and elderly (acting as consultant to other workers), and is now once again a community worker.

'I first met Diana in 1974, when she wrote to the Area Officer about the possibility of setting up a local speech club. At that time I knew very little about speech handicapped people. I had over the years come into contact with a certain number of adults with speech problems, but I hadn't realised that there was anything that could be done which could help them increase their communication. I accepted that what could be done had been done, and really thought no more about it. When we tried to help it was only on the social side.

'I think the same lack of understanding was general. When I asked local social workers if speech handicapped people in Camden presented a general problem, they said no. We did wonder whether a speech club was in fact needed at all, or whether it was all in Diana's mind. However, she impressed us tremendously with her courage and determination, and the example she offered herself of someone who had, with the help of speech therapy, fought back from virtual silence to very adequate communication, and we decided to go ahead.

'She was made the offer of premises from the Guinness Trust Residential Club. (It didn't prove entirely satisfactory, and the speech club was later transferred to Marylebone Institute, but the offer was of great help in actually getting the scheme off the ground.) The club would need transport. Camden laid on a bus to take ten people. Diana found a speech therapist who had trained but retired to have a family, and would be happy to give a three-hour session. The next problem was finance. The transport and premises were both free, but the speech therapist would need to be paid. So I approached the local education authority, ILEA, through the Marylebone Institute, who were very interested and agreed to pay.

'We next needed to find the people to come. I contacted various sources, but the bulk of the referrals came through our queries to hospital speech therapists and social workers. Our speech therapist then went to see each handicapped person individually to explain what was involved. Almost everyone she saw decided to come.

'Once the speech club was started it was obvious it was desperately needed. People came and kept on coming: this isn't always true of support groups we set up. People may come once or twice and then never again, but at the speech club people turned up regularly week after week.

'Diana had been right.'

The problems of starting a speech club* remain the same now as then.

Barbara Deason. 'To set up a speech club the organisers need to find suitable premises, transport, a speech therapist and the money to run it. I can only speak for this area of the country, it may be different elsewhere, but here the education authorities seem more willing to contribute funds than the health and social services, who'll provide transport, but don't see speech therapy as being their concern.'

In other parts of the country, Area Health Authorities may contribute, or the Social Services, Adult Education Centres, or voluntary bodies. (The WRVS was one of the first voluntary organisations to respond to Diana's letter.)

Surprisingly, perhaps, of all the probems, the provision of suitable transport is often the trickiest to solve. Speech handicapped people tend also to be physically handicapped,

* See also page 172

and unable to travel on public transport. Often those concerned have no car, or can no longer drive, or have relatives who are unable to drive. In some areas it may be very difficult to arrange for travel by ambulance. Reliance on voluntary help may be the only solution, but often hard to arrange during the daytime working hours when most speech clubs are held. (The recently introduced mobility allowance will be of help, but falls short of actual costs, especially in remote areas.)

In spite of all the difficulties, the number of speech clubs began slowly to grow.

Diana had – and has – clear ideas as to how these clubs should function.

Her ideal club would meet for a whole day, perhaps in two groups according to speech difficulties. In the morning, one group would have speech therapy while the other would have occupational therapy, art, music, etc. 'Very lot of different things.' After a simple lunch, the groups would switch over. 'Give relatives lovely rest!' Once a month the relatives would come in to meet the others and talk to the speech therapist.

The absolute essential, Diana insists, is the trained speech therapist. Voluntary help is very welcome in all sorts of ways, but as far as recovery of speech is concerned, voluntary help must be informed by and supervised by a professional therapist. And though she doesn't denigrate the social aspect, the emphasis, for Diana, is on 'work work work! No good just games and tea. Work work work . . . a little tea five minutes . . . then work work work!'

INSIDE A SPEECH CLUB

The Camden speech club, started by Diana and Barbara Deason, is held once a week at the Marylebone Institute with Jane Bedingfield as visiting speech therapist. It's for half rather than a full day, but otherwise goes some way towards following her pattern.

Jane Bedingfield was unable to get a grant to train as a speech therapist straight from school, and instead qualified as an SRN at St Bartholomew's. During her fourth year, now with a grant, she began speech therapy training at the Oldrey-Fleming School. She first worked at hospitals in Essex, then after marriage and children moved to the City Literary Institute before taking on the Marylebone speech club.

Jane and the club rely very heavily on the regular help of **Isabel Freedman**, a voluntary worker with Primrose Hill Neighbours Help group, who has been coming here without fail every week for five years. (Up to eighteen months ago the club was also fortunate to have the help of another voluntary worker, Helen Newham.)

The club is held in a large room with comfortable chairs scattered around and original paintings hanging on the walls. A lively group of half a dozen people are sitting round a table absorbed in a game they're playing involving a set of pictures. Another, much quieter group, sits listening intently as a young girl student talks to them.

Jane Bedingfield. 'Peggy Dalton was the real pioneer of speech clubs. She set the whole idea of speech clubs going, and Diana took it up. Diana believed there should be resources for everyone; she was determined to get better herself to help others.

'Although when I first met her – at a branch of the City Lit for the deaf in Bolsover Street – almost all she could say was "but but but", and although she was very depressed, very labile, bursting into tears on the slightest provocation, even then she was very persistent. She also had great compassion for others. When her speech began to improve, if she thought the level was too high for some members of the group, she'd get upset and stay behind afterwards to try to sort things out.

'At that time there were very few speech groups in the country. There were some attached to hospitals, as part of out-patient treatment, but there were restrictions because of the hospital environment, possibilities only for group speech work, and problems over transport. There were day centres outside hospitals for the physically handicapped, where they could meet, play darts, have occupational therapy and so on, but there was nothing similar for the speech-handicapped.

'I think too that it was then generally considered that manual workers were primarily interested in getting their physical condition back, and not really so concerned about speech. I think relatives felt this way too; they were more worried about recovery of movement, about safety, about patients being able to take care of themselves. I disagree with that now, but at that time – ten or eleven years ago – there were so few speech therapists around that many people didn't know what it was all about.

'Peggy Dalton was one of the first to realise the need for much better facilities for all the speech-handicapped, and to press for clubs where they could both meet socially and have therapy. Diana and Barbara Deason did all the background work here; went to see the Principal, had a lot of encouragement from her, and eventually succeeded in putting everything together. I took over after Barbara Deason left.

'The size of the club is restricted by transport problems, nothing else; the Borough of Camden pays to bring ten people in a minibus. A couple are brought by relatives. One manages to make his way by bus. I give a lift to someone who happens to be on my way. Transport is always the difficulty. There are other special classes here for the disabled, such as swimming and keep-fit, but these also depend on people actually getting here.

'I'm paid by ILEA through the Marylebone Institute. The patients themselves pay nothing, except a nominal 5p for biscuits and coffee.

'We get a fairly even mix of men and women. Most have

had strokes, but we also get some with speech difficulties caused by multiple sclerosis or other illnesses affecting the muscles, some Parkinson's, some who've had road accidents. Some people have been coming here for a long while.

'At the moment we have a speech therapy student who has just taken her finals, and one new student. But without Isabel's help this group simply couldn't function. It would be impossible for me to run it on my own; it would be simply a waste of time. Isabel is essential. She's been coming for years and she knows everyone. Without her, I would have to take the group as a whole. It wouldn't work. The differences in levels are too great.

'With Isabel's help we can have two groups. I take the lower one, Isabel the higher-level. When we have students as well, we can split still further. Sometimes we have three or four groups. Sometimes, when we get a new person joining the groups, we can manage a one-to-one session for a while.

'They come between 10 and 10.30. We start by 10.30. We work for three-quarters of an hour, then we have a fifteen-minute break for coffee, and finish by 12.30.

'The main thing is to get people talking: most of them really work at their speech. Every club is different. I don't think this one is necessarily typical. We're not as sociable as some. There isn't the time. Some groups have lots of social activities, with slides and outings and so on, but that wouldn't be much use for our patients. They need the opportunity to talk. We probably see less of their relatives too, since most of the people here come in the minibus. We do have the phone numbers of all the relatives, and when we think it might be helpful we can ask them in and talk to them. It's often a good idea to invite a wife or husband to come and see what's going on, to help them provide some back-up at home.

'I work out a detailed programme beforehand every week.

When I come in, I give Isabel the material for her group, and we have a chat about it if it's necessary. The aim is to give everyone a chance to participate, to stimulate everyone into trying to say something within their capacity. I keep a record of the different stages week by week.

'We try to have something different every Thursday. I don't say today's programme is typical: in fact, I feel perhaps it might be less interesting than other weeks!

'My group does very simple basic things like naming pictures of objects and so on. Isabel has been doing more advanced work using cards with her group.

'Today's programme suggests:
1. Questions for each member of the group.
2. Cockney rhyming slang.
3. A picture quiz.

'Here's a list of small cards I prepared for the first part. Some of them are individual, to match different people's personal tastes. For example: Jim – what is your favourite beer? Anna – what is your favourite food? Tom – what place do you like best in London? Margaret – what is your favourite perfume? While a lot of them are questions for everyone, to stimulate everyone into giving an opinion. What TV programme do you like best? Which time of the year do you prefer?

'This a card for part 2. A list of cockney slang – Band of Hope, bees and honey, boracic lint, and so on – to get them guessing. They did some of this last week, and they enjoyed it. It was a novelty.

'And this is the picture quiz: pictures I've collected from magazines, and a question to ask about each one. Where would you see this man? What kind of flower is this? When did ladies wear dresses like this? Is this made of china or metal? I try to select a variety of pictures and questions to appeal to different tastes.

'For the whole group we have a news quiz on the week's affairs. Anything from "What happened to Canada's DC9 the other day?" to "Where is Liz Taylor at the moment?" to "Have gold prices gone up or down?"

'So Isabel has the work mapped out, but she follows it using her own discretion.'

Isabel Freedman. 'I only use what Jane gives me, but I know all the group individually, so I can give the questions the right emphasis. I know what interests each particular person. I try to get each one to say something. And I make jokes – I try to get them to laugh. We can be pretty noisy sometimes!

'They enjoy coming. Some have been with us ever since the club started, some are new, some come only now and again. It makes it easier for them when they see how many others are in the same boat. I think most of them gain confidence. Some make real progress . . . some don't seem to move.

'I helped one of my group write a piece for his church. He's really proud of it; it's made quite a difference to him. I think maybe it's the only really constructive thing I've done here!

'Progress depends a lot on the individual. There's one man here, a new one, now he's *determined* to get better. He tries to be independent all the time. If he can possibly do something, he does it.'

Those involved in the running of speech clubs are in no doubt of their value.

Jane Bedingfield. 'We feel the club is very well worth while. For some of these people it may be almost the only chance in the week they get to meet and talk to others. We're all behind Diana in her efforts to promote speech clubs so that many more can benefit.'

Barbara Deason. 'What's important is that they give handicapped people the feeling that someone believes it worth while trying to help them, after the hospital has given them up. It gives hope to relatives, too. I've seen them work. The one we started, when I first went no one said a word. They just sat around. It was the same week after week. Then I didn't go for a while, and when I went back some time later someone looked up and said, "Hello!" I was surprised and delighted. Everyone was obviously improving, and enjoying it as well.'

Later, in 1975, Diana described on the radio programme PM what her speech clubs could do:

My dear, and lovely, and lovely people, can't speak a word perhaps, little and a little, and a little, come up, it's lovely *to see them progressing.*

11 A campaign for 'other people'

From this time on Diana was to devote most of her time to the promotion and encouragement of speech clubs; and to the cause of speech therapy in general.

None of this would have been possible without the support of her friends and the practical day-to-day help of what she calls her 'scribes'. Her 'scribe-system' began shortly after she left the CMRC. One of their voluntary workers, 'Blanchy,' Miss V.T.Blanchfield, went to visit Diana to help her with letters about her financial affairs. Diana soon realised how much this kind of help enlarged her possibilities, and bit by bit a list of volunteers was built up.

Mary Law. 'There's one thing we couldn't be more grateful for and couldn't manage without, and that's the willingness of so many people to give up their time to come and visit Diana and write all her many letters for her. We sometimes have four or five scribes a day. We offer them coffee or sherry – I take care of a lot of that. I say to her, "You make the proposals and I make the disposals!"

'All sorts of people come. Through friends, the WRVS, Westminster and Camden Councils, or her colleagues in the British Council. For example, there's one who's a secretary in the City, a solicitor who's Swiss, a nurse, a Welsh girl, a young doctor, a Roman Catholic Irish gentlewoman, a young girl who's not much more than a school-girl. Between them they make all the difference to her ability to communicate and carry on her campaign to help other people.'

To Diana her scribes are a vital link with the outside world. As she says herself about the letters she wants to send: 'In my mind lovely, but coming out . . . !'

Moira Tighe and Betty Giles are only two of many who take what Diana wants to say, capture the sense in words, and pin these to paper.

Moira Tighe was an author's secretary for most of her working life. She started at twenty-five working for F. Tennyson Jesse (author of the detective classic *A Pin to See the Peepshow, The Lacquer Lady* and many others). She travelled extensively with her and her husband, H.M.Harwood (who worked on the script for Garbo's *Queen Christina*); staying in such exotic places as the Riviera (where she played golf with Somerset Maugham), Hollywood, Burma, Ceylon and Rio. She also worked as Secretary for the Court of Appeal in Nairobi. She made a gradual retirement as arthritis became a problem, and went to Camden Council to seek suitable voluntary work.

'Since words had been my trade all my life, I was looking for some way to make use of my experience. When they told me about Diana, scribing for her sounded like something I could do. I'm good at thinking myself into another person's place.

'Diana tells me what sort of terms she's on with whoever she's writing to. She gives me the gist of what she wants to say, and then I put it into fluent English. I do know shorthand, but I don't use it with Diana. It's much more a question of finding out about relationships, so I can write the sort of letter Diana wants to send; whether to be chatty, or more formal. Sometimes I can be a bit foxed about what she wants to say, and we'll have quite a session trying to get it straight, but mostly we're on the same wavelength. We happen to have a lot in common. I'm from Ireland, like her family, and I talk about Dublin and the old days to her mother. I'm a great admirer of them both: they're survivors.'

Betty Giles is a personal secretary in the Civil Service who has been one of Diana's scribes since 1972.

'I saw an advertisement for volunteers from the WRVS in *Miss London* or *Girl*. It said something like "If you have a few moments to spare come to a special evening." I couldn't go, but I rang up, and I went along to the WRVS and had an interview. I said that I'd be no good at hospital visiting – I'd sit there getting more upset than the patients – so they suggested that I might be able to help Diana. I went along one evening, and the whole thing snowballed from there.

'I go every Wednesday after work. I don't do any short-hand; it isn't necessary. Sometimes I write letters there, sometimes I just make notes and then type the letters later at home. There are times when I feel tired beforehand, but after I leave Diana I always feel I've done something worth while.'

With people like these to help her, Diana set to work on her two-pronged publicity campaign.

For her speech clubs, she responded to all the queries which came to her as a result of ever-increasing publicity. Enquirers were sent a questionnaire asking for information about the availability of speech therapy, help given, provision of transport etc; suggestions for the organisation of a club and ideas for activities. She was also prepared to travel and talk to groups at churches, schools or voluntary organisations; to do anything or go anywhere to help her cause. As she puts it: 'I want to be able to talk about other people . . . Other people haven't got a chance.'

'I WANT SPEECH THERAPY TO HAVE BIG PRESS'

At the same time that Diana was promoting speech clubs, she began seriously campaigning for the cause of speech therapy itself.

The time was favourable. The 1972 report of the Committee on Speech Therapy Services (set up in 1969), generally referred to as the Quirk report, disclosed a situation where an estimated 40,000 adults were in need of speech therapy; far too few speech therapists were being trained; and pay – compared with parallel professions – was low.

Before the Quirk report, few – apart from the handicapped themselves and those dealing directly with them – were aware of the important role speech therapists had to play, and of the obstacles in their path. As Professor Quirk put it in a radio programme: 'When you think of the powerful and well-organised dental services, devoted to helping people to chew, it is quite devastating to think how little our society has done to build up and sustain the profession whose job it is to help people to *talk* and so to participate in man's most important attribute: his ability to use words.'

While speech therapy was clearly vital, it was not at that time accepted as such even by many who were closely involved.

As the Quirk report stated: 'There is a striking contrast between the value attached to the speech therapist's work and the ignorance, in many quarters, of the complexity, range and difficulty of that work; between the eagerness of employers to recruit speech therapists and the poor working conditions offered, between the readiness to enlist the speech therapist's help and the reluctance, in some professions, to accept her as a colleague upon equal terms.'

To press the need for more and better paid speech therapists Diana wrote, and wrote again, to every source of support she could find. Her files bulge with letters to the press, TV, radio, the DHSS, Universities, Departments of Audiology, Ministers of Health, RADAR, individual speech therapists; and above all with letters to Members of Parliament.

I used to be Conservative. Now I am for speech therapists, and for all *parties. All the time writing to MPs and the House of Lords. I'm* very *impatient!*

The pace was too slow for Diana. But the knowledge that the number of speech clubs *was* growing, that gradually more therapists were being trained and their pay increased, helped to keep her crusading spirit alive through the trials of the next few years.

12　Physical set-backs

Diana's work was to be hampered, at times for considerable periods, by various bouts of ill health.

I had three fits. One bad one at the Wolfson. Then a fainting fit at home. My mother found me on the floor. Another in Daphne Stafford's. I was taken to Guildford Hospital.

Daphne Stafford still recalls this last occasion as 'a terrible shock.'

'It was the first time she'd come to stay with me since her stroke. No one had warned me about possible hazards.

'That first evening she was in cracking form. Then suddenly from another room I heard a crash. I went in and found her on the floor. I thought she'd had another stroke. I eventually got the doctor and she went to hospital, where I was told that she'd had a major epileptic fit, and not the first one. I had had no idea that this might happen. Suppose she'd had her fit at the top of the stairs?

'I've been told since that a fit is a hazard for a stroke patient, especially someone highly intelligent trying to get back to normal too fast. If I'd been warned, perhaps I would have recognised it. She was so . . . over-geared when she came. Even when I went to the hospital, she had everyone roaring with laughter.'

Joan Ellams cautions, however, of the need to take the overall view.

'A stroke patient *may* have a fit, but the possibility is unpredictable. It depends basically on where the situation of the brain damage is. If it is in such a place that a fit is a possibility, then the likelihood increases in stress situations; but many in stress situations may never have a fit at all because the brain damage is not such as to cause it.

'Even when a patient does have a fit, this may be the only one and never repeated. Sometimes doctors are reluctant to put patients on anti-convulsants unless there seems no alternative. It's also important not to put too much emphasis on the fit. Patients' relatives can become over-protective, so that they're prevented from doing anything and going anywhere because of the possibility, however slight, of another fit. It's a question of balance, of what is best. We're dealing always in shades of grey.'

Diana was prescribed anti-convulsants and had no further fits, apart from what she describes as:

Lots of little ones once a month. Very slight fainting fits, but not right out. Perhaps sick or not. Maybe to do with no periods?

IN-PATIENT AT THE MIDDLESEX

Diana then went on to suffer from a succession of illnesses, not directly connected with her stroke, which caused her great pain and necessitated long weeks of in-patient treatment at the Middlesex Hospital: an attack of renal-tubular acidosis with, simultaneously, myxoedema (under-active thyroid), which led to a three-month stay; then trouble with her right leg, leading to a further six-week stay; and towards the end of 1976 a problem with her good leg, which eventually improved.

Diana faced these times with great courage; and, as those in the Middlesex who came into contact with her can testify, made use of her time there to further the understanding of stroke patients and the cause of speech therapy.

Dr JDHS, 'part of the brickwork' at the Middlesex, is a General Physician and Senior Lecturer who trained here, took various house-jobs in other hospitals, including Hammersmith, spent a period in the States, was asked to return and has stayed at the Middlesex ever since.

'Diana had an obscure kidney malfunction which affected her bones, eventually diagnosed as renal tubular acidosis. She had a lot of pain.

'Anyway, we managed to put things right, but it was a long process, and required great fortitude on Diana's part. She only slowly began to realise that she would be all right, and it took time for her bones to heal.

'Then she had problems too with her right leg. There was never any question of cancer, but I was afraid that it might develop into a prolonged infection which could have crippled her. Some while ago I would have been gloomy about the function of that right leg, but fortunately it turned out much better than at one time I had feared.

'Diana of course still takes a large quantity of pills every day. Most of these are not drugs, but mineral supplements, which she has to take and continue to take in large quantities.

'When I first met her, shortly after she had written her letter to the *Daily Telegraph*, she was already a good speaker, and had begun to start the first of her speech clubs.

'I suppose it's true to say that I do have considerable sympathy for people with speech problems. As a general physician I have encountered a variety of speech problems; and, because of Diana, when the possibility came up of expanding speech therapy facilities, I did promote the cause of speech therapy rather more than other contenders for the space. Now speech therapy is very soundly based here.

'I've also gone out of my way to expose students to her. When she comes and speaks before a large group, her speech gets better. It's unusual, but for Diana her speech actually improves under this sort of pressure. When she is trying to put her point, when she feels she is being really useful, she becomes more and not less articulate.

'One of the difficulties speech therapy faces at present is the lack of hard data on its effectiveness, but there is no doubt at all of its value on humanitarian grounds. Oddly enough – and I've never mentioned this to Diana, and I don't believe I've ever thought about it before in this context – but I had a speech problem myself when I was younger. In my childhood and youth I could hardly get a word out edgeways. When I was seventeen I saw a speech therapist called Amy Swallow. She was terrific. She used to make me recite poems for hours on end. I'm sure that she helped me a lot. . . .'

Diana spent most of her time at the Middlesex in the Queen Alexandra Ward with Sister Heather Griffin.

Heather Griffin trained at the Middlesex, did midwifery in Portsmouth and Cirencester, then returned to the Middlesex as night sister; and came to the Queen Alexandra Ward (a general medical ward) in 1968, where she has been ever since. 'I suppose the Middlesex is my home from home.'

'I believe that Diana was under the rheumatologists first, then when it was discovered that the pain in her leg might be due to a bio-chemical disturbance she was transferred here.

'I felt she was nervous about coming to another hospital.

She'd spent so much time in hospitals that she was frightened of becoming institutionalised. She was determined not to lose her independence. From the moment she got here she wouldn't let us do anything. She even insisted on taking baths on her own. We were all astonished that she was so independent with such disabilities.

'It was good for our nurses to see someone with a stroke who could cope. Mostly we get people just after they've had their stroke, and they're very dependent. Nurses are trained to do things for their patients. It goes against their training to let people struggle with something, and anyway they haven't the time to wait for two hours while someone does up one button, but it's good for them to realise that this isn't necessarily the best way of helping.

'As far as Diana's speech goes, once we'd got on to the same wavelength we felt she could communicate 100 per cent. Getting used to talking to her has helped our nurses to be less diffident about listening to people with speech difficulties. Young nurses in particular are often shy when they first arrive in the ward. They tend to go to people who are easy to talk to, and then they hide there. Diana has helped them to get over this.

'The moment she arrived she broke down the barrier that's often felt between nurses and patients. She used to go across and greet the nurses as soon as they came through the door. She took them over, made them feel part of a family.

'I must confess I had to fight hard against the impulse to finish her conversation. I'm afraid I may still do it sometimes! I know it must be infuriating. I remember when she first came, she might only want to say something like "I have a pain in my leg," but because she was so slow, we'd try to jump in to say, "Is it in your head?" "Is it in your arm?" and in the end it might take half an hour, whereas if we'd just had the patience to wait she'd have got it across much more quickly. She knew exactly what she wanted to say. The more we tried to fill in, the more upset she got. We did learn in the end!

'Diana's improving all the time. The longest we have a patient in the ward is six months or so, and progress is so slow that often we think there isn't any. But we only see Diana at intervals, so that each time I see her I appreciate that there's been a change. It's an important point. Nurses, like other people, expect to see progress much more rapidly than is possible.

'I'm entirely in support of her efforts to improve understanding among the medical profession as well as outside. The practice of speech therapy depends very much on the backing it gets from the top. I think in some cases consultants don't understand and perhaps don't want to understand. I believe there may be an element of fear in it. Faced with speech disabilities, few doctors can *do* anything. The knowledge that they can't makes them uneasy. I think sometimes they're inclined to brush it all aside.

'We don't have enough speech therapists. On the wards we could make more use of those we have if we could get the nurses together to watch what the therapist is doing, so we could do our best to continue the exercises and make sure we're doing the right thing. Sometimes we're not. For example, some patients have difficulty in swallowing. Now, speech therapists show us that throat muscles can be trained more easily to cope with solids than with fluids: yet nurses are trained to give fluids. Where patients are unable to swallow fluids, we may resort to feeding them through nasal tubes simply to keep them alive, when in fact this might not be necessary at all, and by retraining the muscles and giving them solids we could enable them to return far more quickly to a normal way of life.

'So in many ways Diana is a very *practical* example to all the nurses here. We often see her. She walks here from her home, and she always pops up to have a chat and hand out her latest leaflets and bits of information. It's good for our morale as well. Mostly, when patients leave, we never see them again. When they come back for check-ups, it takes so much energy, and some of them still have such difficulty in moving around, that they understandably don't want to take the extra effort to get up here. When Diana comes, it gives us a boost.'

Diana's friends continued to rally round her. Anne Handley-Derry recalls accompanying her to the Middlesex on several of her out-patient visits.

'It could be embarrassing at times. I was there purely in a supportive role, to help her communicate if there were problems, or so I could explain afterwards to Mrs Law if it seemed there might be difficulties.

'To start with it was a bit awkward not being a relative, but eventually I was accepted as being helpful.

'Now Diana goes to the Middlesex only once every three months for a routine check-up. If she's at all worried I go too, and go through her list of pills and medicines with her.'

Today Diana feels her health is good; she takes with aplomb the battery of tablets which control her condition. For her tendency to fits, 3 phenobarbitone a day; for her kidneys, 1 spiromolactome, 4 slow K, 8 potassium bi-carbonate, $\frac{1}{2}$ phosphate sandoz per day; for her thyroid trouble, I thyroxine a day; plus 5 diazepam (to prevent spasms in her right arm and leg) daily, and 1 Mogadon and 2 painkillers only when required. In addition Diana takes a vitamin D tablet and one multivitamin daily.

She still has trouble and sometimes pain in her legs. 'My good leg gets cramped. My bad leg and arm go into spasms in heavy traffic.' She herself believes that, because she made a deliberate choice to concentrate all her energies on speaking, her arm and leg are both weaker than they might otherwise have been. If others choose instead to concentrate on physical recovery, that's where their improvement will take place.

If there was indeed a choice, Diana is sure she made the right one.

13 Fight for mobility

Diana's energies were 'squandered' through these years on what Mrs Law describes as 'the car saga'.

Diana herself saw her struggle with bureaucracy as not a personal but a general issue. 'I fight always for others.' If she, with her organising ability and persistence, with family and friends to help, with scribes to write for her, could so singularly fail to get her rights, what chance had those even more handicapped than herself?

Her efforts to get the Invacar to which she was entitled began seriously in February 1974. Already at the end of 1968, at her check-up at the Wolfson, it had been suggested (as Dr A-M T reports) that Diana should consider getting in touch with the BSM to start driving again, as her reaction time on the simulator was within the normal range.

However, it was not until after her year at Camden, her continued improvement, and the publication of her *Daily Telegraph* letter that Diana felt ready to apply for an invalid car. In August 1973, at a CMRC check-up, she discussed the possibility of driving again, and in February 1974 she made an official application.

The prospect of being once more truly mobile meant a great deal to her. Before her stroke, Diana had driven herself all over the country and was always ready to take planes and trains. Now, it was a problem getting anywhere unless she could walk – very slowly – or a friend could take her.

Mary Law. 'She tried to go by bus once, and tube once, but it didn't work. The escalators are impossible. She moves too slowly getting on and off, and the bus platforms are too high. It's the same with taxis; the step's too high. We use Abbey cars, but we can't afford to do it too often. It's so expensive now.'

A car of her own would mean freedom; and the possibility of devoting more time to her cause.

Delivery was originally promised around November 1974. There followed five years of frustration.

Diana's file headed 'CAR' contains over 140 separate bits of paper: forms, letters, replies, omissions, copies sent from one person and department to another. Those writing to Diana are courteous, thoughtful, desirous to help, but handicapped by the splitting of responsibilities between different departments. Arrangements are made but upset by some break in the chain of communication. A car is eventually delivered, but to the wrong place. Modifications are made, but the wrong ones. The ambulance due to take Diana for a driving lesson is cancelled, so the test is missed. Appointments are made with only two or three days' notice, so they can't be kept.

Diana's illnesses over the years caused breaks in the sequences, which didn't help; but her efforts to get back to where she was before the latest set-back weren't helped by an accumulation of niggling details.

She was not taken to the disabled persons' entrance at County Hall. The incorrect sum was sent as a refund by the transport department. The wrong badge was issued. And so on: all small things, but each wasting energy, each involving yet another letter to be written and the answer noted and filed.

A letter written by a scribe for Diana in May 1975 is typical of her correspondence.

1. Received (the car) on Wednesday, 14 May 1975. Delivery taken by Mr L, not by myself; although I was at home the man who delivered it failed to inform me.

2. I telephoned DHSS Euston Appliance Centre the following day, and gave the reference number. I pointed out that it had been parked on the east side of HS by the synagogue.

3. The car was then removed by C Motors to the west side of the street.

4. The car cannot however be used:
   a) because the wrong key was left with it.
   b) more important, it is fitted for driving with the right hand or both hands, not left hand only. I originally made it clear that I can drive *only* with the left hand and foot.

5. The fire appliance is also on the wrong side; the instruments are also unsuited to driving with the left hand only.

6. There was no carrier's receipt; according to the letter reference dated 15 May this should have been returned 'Not examined' but there was no such receipt to return.

7. My name is incorrectly spelt on the letter mentioned in 6 above and on the certificate of motor insurance.

8. Following rain the *inside* of the car was very wet.

9. The driver/deliverer opened the car with his key. I was unable to close the door because it is very stiff.

Following Diana's heart-felt request ('*Please* please help me') the car was finally correctly modified. It took over four more years.

Her problems were still not over.

A letter dated 13.8.79 comments: 'I am *fed up* with all the problems with this car. They are as follows:

1. No petrol was in the car, so my instructor and I went to get some, but the petrol cap was so rusted to the car that it took ages to get it off.

2. I cannot get into the car from the nearside but I do not know the explanation for this.

3. While driving, the steering handle hits my knee, which is very painful, and I therefore think that the seat must be in the wrong position for me. . . .

I beg you to do something quickly, because as I said before I'm *fed up* with being unable to drive.

But, by the end of 1979, Diana finally and reluctantly decided, after her prolonged struggle, to give up the idea of a car. On December 12th she wrote to apply instead for special mobility allowance.

It was a disappointment.

There were so many places to go to, so many people to see, to further her cause. Though the allowance was a help, with transport costs so high and increasing all the time, she felt she was still far from having the mobility she needed.

It was 'back to the drawing-board.'

14   Osborne – an oasis

Diana's mainstay throughout this fruitful but arduous period was undoubtedly her twice-yearly visits to Osborne, The King Edward VII's Convalescent Home for Officers in Queen Victoria's house in the Isle of Wight. At first taxing, her later visits were – and are – sources of refreshment and encouragement.

Mary Law. 'Osborne means a great deal to her. She goes there twice a year. She meets people like herself, and she can enjoy the sort of social life she loves right through the evenings.'

My routine is but 1,2,3,4,5,6 – 6.45 tea is served. Sister on night duty bringing the tea and lots of pills. At 7 wash myself. 8 o'clock the pool. The pool is hot pool. The valet comes for me in the wheelchair. I all ready too. My bathing dress is there and dressing gown is Osborne but towelling. In the cold. Ordinary person walk down, but me the passage. I'm going into the cold. In two minutes very cold. In very cold weather I have a blanket on.

Now I walk into the pool. But two years I have to help the valet and instructor and extra men to help me down. And hose very big hose very strong. 1,2,3,4,5,6,7, eight persons in pool and instructor. And mixed – women and men.

But one half hour but going back to change my bathing

dress and take it off in my room and hang it up to dry in hot press.

But to have my breakfast in bed. But too much struggle dressing. But I like it! Toast and coffee.

Taylor very nice man. Fifteen minutes. 'The torture chamber.' The gymnast a lot of very horrible tortures go on! I like it enormously.

OT too busy half-day only. All the very crippled people in the morning.

At twelve going to the golf club. Ten minutes going. A Guinness. Walk back.

In the afternoon I go down to the beach but by car. The beach car available or someone else. The tea . . . Guests allowed in dining-room at tea but no other time.

I play golf but putting in the grounds after tea but the dinner is 7 o'clock but you must be changed. Drinking hours very restricted. 6.20 – 6.50. But wine in dining-room. The maids have the lovely purple dress, long white aprons and a hat. Lovely silver cups. Serving all the time. Waitress comes and serves you.

Evening I have very good time in billiards room. Play funny game – one hand billiard bowls. Another game I always champion. I like shove ha'penny. Dominoes. Golf – putting. Bagatelle.

Competition each week. In each game six prizes. Friday dinner night. House governor and wife and lots of people from London come and visit. Prizes afterwards. Always win. Row of books. Good to get to know one another.

Always talk to new people. Monday . . . Wednesday . . . Friday . . . going away and coming back. Lots of people not expecting lots of corridors and lame people and very thing . . . And I show them around.

Mmmmm . . . Saturday the same.

Sunday to church. Whippingham all the time Victoriana. In the basement of Osborne have a chapel too. Clergyman

*very nice, but I have to wash my hair on Sunday, stay in
bed, bath, washing, and I can't go to church!*

*I like to stay in the grounds, but always before the war
I had a lovely house Cowes week. All the island I know
very well.*

*I like Osborne. The trees and shrubs are very special. The
birds and the foxes. And squirrels are* red *squirrels. I like
to see the sea.*

*One thing is absent. Speech therapy! I have tried. But
speech therapist in island now one year there. But I first
speaking no speak at all!*

*Meet all the time different and the same people. Very
good.*

*Like Camden. All the staff . . . the gardeners, the house
governor, everyone. All the staff . . . the patients are the
first and the staff second.*

HOME, HOSPITAL, HOTEL

Osborne offers Diana – and others like her – days full of
planned activity, the company of people in similar circumstances, the chance to participate, all in a highly organised
and harmonious setting.

The first stone of Osborne House itself was laid by
Queen Victoria and her husband in 1845. Prince Albert
was reminded by the view across the Solent on a fine day
of the Bay of Naples, and Osborne is a nineteenth century
version of a Palladian palazzo. The State Apartments, now
open to the public (and free to visitors at the Convalescent
Home) are much lighter and brighter than the word 'Vic-
torian' conjures up. The colours are clear and summery.
Much of the furniture recalls the eighteenth century and
pre-dates the elaborate taste of later years. The paintings
and photos and souvenirs of a long reign and longer life
fill the rooms but without overwhelming them. The same
sense of lightness and space – and the close ties with a still-
recent past – spill over into the King Edward VII's Home

which, since 1904, has occupied the former Household Wing.

The patients' rooms are spacious, high-ceilinged, painted in delicate pastels with tall gilt-edged light-reflecting mirrors. Rich red carpets muffle footsteps in the long high corridors, hung with Winterhalter princesses, photos and sepia drawings of Queen Victoria's enormous sprawling family, paintings of ships, favourite dogs, and historical events. Classical plaster heads gaze down into stairwells, the brass knobs twinkle with loving care not lacquer, and even the flower arrangements recall nineteenth-century still-lifes.

Outside, Italianate gardens stretch out on all sides in a succession of smooth lawns, shaved hedges, urn-topped walls, pergolas and loggias and fountains and flower beds; and then, on the north side, give way to meadows and a stretch of woodland spilling down on to the private beach where once Queen Victoria went down into the sea in a bathing-machine. ('I thought it was delightful until I put my head under the water, when I thought I would have stifled.')

The gardens and the beach are open at any time to Osborne patients. Some, like Diana, enjoy the birds and wildlife which find sanctuary here. Others sit and read in the sheltered spots, while more active visitors can enjoy croquet, golf, or even sailing.

The atmosphere is of hope, tranquillity, and a complete severing from the cares and preoccupations of everyday life. There is a suspension of time here which can be healing in itself. All – porters, valets, maids, therapists, nurses – seem happy to dedicate themselves to restoring life and vitality to those who come here: many have been working at Osborne for ten, fifteen, twenty years. Once here the visitor can for a brief period allow himself or herself to relax and creatively concentrate on mending body and spirit.

Originally, those who came to the King Edward VII's Convalescent Home had to be serving officers who had been injured or had contracted illnesses during their years of service. Now, however, it's open to anyone who is serving or has ever served as an officer of the Armed Services, to serving or retired members of the Civil Service, or to their spouses. Moreover, anyone coming for a convalescent holiday may now bring his or her spouse. There is only one qualification: anyone wishing to come must be fit enough to attend the dining-room for all meals.

Diana has been going to Osborne now since 1969. Her stays here are not only high-spots in an otherwise hardworking life, but a chance for her mother to feel free to visit other members of her family. Most visitors to Osborne come far less frequently; but whatever the illness, or whether they come once or make repeated visits, each visitor can be sure of individual care and a lively, participating interlude.

THE DAILY ROUND

For most visitors, life at Osborne follows a settled pattern. Admissions are phased over three days — Mondays, Wednesdays and Fridays — so that individual attention can be given.

Diana, like all patients, sees the house governor and nursing staff soon after her arrival. Medical notes are communicated only to the house governor; the nursing staff are responsible for the maintenance of the often highly complicated drug regimes which differ for each patient. Osborne staff stay for years, and so can see the progress of those patients who — like Diana — return visit after visit.

One of the house governors. He works in the room where Queen Victoria used to sit and listen to her ministers (ranged in the room alongside) reading out the contents of the latest bills; under an elegant ceiling with magnificent plaster work picked out in gold leaf on bands of colour, lit by a multi-coloured candelabra of Bavarian glass, entwined with lilies and convolvulus. Visitors who come to consult him have the choice of sitting on either Queen Victoria's own chair or Prince Albert's, while they rest their feet on the original carpet, lustrous as ever.

'Diana has been here nineteen times. I've been here for her last nine visits. I've seen her make immense progress, specially in the last five years. When I first arrived her speech was only a series of "but . . . but . . . buts." Now she can communicate well.

'She's progressed emotionally too. During her last visits, since her stay at the Middlesex, she's been quite different. Less threatening, less demanding. She used to be a very emotional lady right from her first entry. If she'd had a good foot she'd have stamped it. She was very demanding on all the staff – the kitchen people, cleaners, valets, everyone. Though of course everyone could sympathise with her frustration; she has a very good intellect but was unable to communicate.

'I know Diana would like a resident speech therapist, but we could never justify one here. Only a very small proportion of patients have speech problems. We do get stroke patients who are even more handicapped than Diana was, but they're a tiny minority. We do occasionally have patients straight from hospital who can only grunt, but I still see our primary concern, in the short time they're here, to improve their locomotion. Most of them are elderly – younger patients tend to go to Headley Court or Epsom. Some of them may be responsible for another elderly person, or even nursing an aging relative. So I see mobility as being of prime importance.'

'In addition, many elderly people never speak much anyway, especially if they live alone. That's one of the reasons we organise these games every night. You can't play them in total silence. That's also why we have elevenses, afternoon tea, pre-meal drinks and a last-minute cup of tea at night. It's possible for people to sit down and eat a meal and go away without saying a word, but they can't do that with a cup of hot tea. It helps to get people back into the habit of speaking. I've had many visitors come and thank me for the chance of participating in a social life again. Of course that's one of the things Diana loves here. She's very good at a lot of the games. I'm always awarding her prizes.'

'In theory we can take fifty-one visitors at a time; in practice this is more than I like. We can often take people even at very short notice, so we're in a position to help with patients coming directly from hospital after a sudden emergency.

'We do circulate details of Osborne very widely, but I know a lot of the information simply never gets through to those who would be interested. Quite a high proportion of people convalescing here come because they know someone who knows someone who came, or a relative told them – not because they were encouraged by their doctor or welfare officer. I feel too that perhaps some people who hear about us without knowing any details think that we only welcome generals and admirals, but anyone who comes here can see it's not at all like that. Considering how extensive the Civil Service is, and how many people served as officers in the war and afterwards, a really high proportion of the population must be eligible to come. Especially now that we take spouses – whether they come for the treatment themselves or just to accompany their husbands or wives.

'There are other convalescent homes, of course. The King Edward VII Trust will give details of others like ours. Trade unions run homes as well. A lot of these do have a very closed membership. It's a question of asking around. Depending on circumstances, a welfare officer may be able to help, or a GP, or even a local library.

'One particularly important aspect of convalescence is that we can give *families* a break. When someone comes here after a stroke, like Diana, or a road accident, or perhaps someone crippled with arthritis, their relatives can breathe a sigh of relief, knowing that our patients are getting excellent care – and we hope enjoying themselves as well –

while for a short time they themselves can get away and have some of the pressure taken off. We appreciate that caring for some of our visitors can be a full-time job, and we like to know we're helping to take some of the strain.'

Betty Denny came to Osborne in 1967 after her training at Hammersmith Hospital and working in Canada and Australia. She left there on her marriage in 1972, then returned for a brief spell of night duty after her husband's death.

'I was Senior Sister when Diana came to Osborne on her very first visit. She came as an ex-Major. We used to get mostly service people then; now I think Osborne gets more civil servants.

'She was very bad then. Very low. She had hardly any words. She could say "My dear!" and "But!" She got very frustrated. It must have been dreadful for her, wanting to get things done and not being able to get it across. She could only walk a little – it was a struggle for her. She cried a lot. That's one of the things about strokes. It makes people emotional.

'But even then there was something unusual about her. She was never self-conscious. And she always tried.'

Una Gavin trained at Harefield during the war, then worked at every kind of nursing in many different parts of the world: Ireland, the United States (Boston, New Plymouth, San Francisco), New Zealand. She came to Osborne as an ordinary sister, and then took over from Sister Betty Denny as sister-in-charge. She 'loves it here. I like the life, the work, the feeling that we're helping people, seeing people improve as they come back again.'

'We don't get many stroke patients; perhaps an average of three or four at a time. Diana, when she first came, was among the most severely handicapped.

'She was never an easy patient. She went through a bad frustration phase at the beginning. If she didn't get what she

wanted, heaven help us all! But we could cope. We had the
staff and the time to cope. There'd be weeping sessions if
she couldn't get her own way. "I want a room!" when she
wanted a particular room, and not the room we'd given her.
She wanted *her* way. She wouldn't accept reason. She could
only see things from her side. But we could reassure her and
help her through it. We did our best to accommodate her
and cope with her tears. Then she'd come out of the tears
and laugh. "Sorry!"

'She always did everything she could. After her first visits,
she brought her little washboard with her so she could wash
out her smalls with one hand.

'And she's always cheerful with the other patients. She
makes a point of recognising them. Involving them. She
always wants to be doing things.

'Medicine says that most of the improvement after a
stroke comes in the first two years, even in the first year;
this hasn't been so with Diana. Sheer determination plus
her speech therapy have kept her progressing. Nobody could
have imagined from those early days how far she would
go, so who can say what will happen in the future?'

Constance Offord. 'Diana has made a great improvement
in just the last two years. Three years or so ago she was
clinically very upset. She wasn't her usual Diana self. Something was wrong with her metabolism – nothing to do with
her stroke. Rather, there was something on top, over and
above her stroke. After Diana's treatment at the Middlesex
Hospital, the change has been quite dramatic. She's much
more cheerful, more settled in herself.

'Having seen so many ill people, I've always said "Anything else but a stroke." For so many people a stroke becomes a life sentence. Diana hasn't allowed hers to do that
to her. Yet, with someone like Diana, you constantly have
the two thoughts side by side. The waste of someone who
was so gifted and could have done so much. And the

courage and determination which has made her fight back against so many handicaps to be the campaigning person she is today.'

Diana's day starts with morning tea brought to her large high-ceilinged room; then a pre-breakfast visit to the hydrotherapy pool. For someone in a wheelchair – Diana without her calliper – this involves a short trip in the open pushed by one of the valets.

Cyril Easterbrook. 'I've been a valet here for fourteen and a half years; my colleague, John Hawkins, who's just retired, was here for twenty-seven. We look after the patients in every possible way, except for medically.

'John or I used to take Miss Law for her treatment every time. She liked to be wrapped up in a blanket just so, her feet all tucked in, no little gaps for drafts. Once she got down to the pool, we only lifted her in those first times when it was absolutely necessary. As soon as she could manage, she did it on her own.

'She was always very independent, Miss Law. She does all her packing and unpacking herself. She asks for her suitcases three or four days before she goes, and they're always ready in time.

'There's never any self-pity. Never a complaint. She could have been in a wheelchair for evermore, but she's really worked at getting better. I know other patients find her an inspiration. They've told me so.

'She really enjoys the pool. Always pleased to go in, always sorry to come out.'

The pool is only small – nine feet by twelve – with seats, bars and trapezes. It gurgles with constantly changing water which is kept at a constant temperature of 95°F. The room is enclosed, green and snug; it feels and sounds like a Turkish bath.

After her session, Diana dresses too slowly to be able to breakfast in the dining-room; most of the other visitors arrive there promptly at 8.30.

Rather as on a cruise-ship, meals – and snacks – establish a framework for the day. Breakfast at 8.30, luncheon at 1 pm, tea at 4.30 pm and dinner at 7 pm.

The dining-room is formal, with long polished tables set with starched white linen runners. On one side are high floor-to-ceiling windows, on the other a marble mantelpiece and old oil lamps with dark green shades. Massive silver cups gleam from the table centres. sporting trophies presented by long-ago regiments in far-away places; the tea-urns sit on heavy silver trays; the starched white napkins fold into shining silver rings engraved with ER VII.

There are no fixed places. Patients may sit where they choose and where there is space, but all are expected to be punctual and not encouraged to linger past a certain point.

Visitors must fetch and pour out their own cups of tea at breakfast and tea, but the well-cooked meals themselves are served by cheerful maids in light maroon dresses with starched white aprons and caps. Breakfast: cereal, a different cooked dish each day, an individual rack of toast. Lunch: a main dish with vegetables and a light pudding. Tea: bread and butter, jam and Marmite, home-baked cakes. Dinner: three courses, followed by coffee. At lunch bottled drinks only are served, but at dinner patients may also buy glasses of wine – though only for themselves and not for others.

After breakfast, patients separate to take part in their individually designed programmes.

While Diana is dressing, those who are able go off for a general session in the Victoria Hall, used both for recreation and exercises. Big windows look out on to the formal garden. Footballs are piled by the large marble-and-tile fireplace. Brass finger plates and knobs twinkle in the light coming through the stained glass borders in the windows.

Here, and in the 'torture chamber', lined with fine wooden exercise equipment dating from the thirties (due to be retired now that lighter substitutes have replaced it), Diana and her fellow-visitors go through prescribed exercises under the supervision of Ted Taylor, physiotherapist, and Bill Hepplewhite, remedial gymnast.

Ted Taylor trained as a physiotherapist in the RAF, working with patients from RAF families of from six weeks to sixty. He's been working at Osborne since 1969, and so has been seeing Diana ever since her first visit here.

'When she first came, Diana's speech was very bad. I could understand her, but her vocabulary was very small indeed. When she first came, she couldn't get her calliper on and off herself. Now she does everything herself.

'I do the gentler exercises, and more individual therapy than Bill. With me, three people make a group. I never have more.

'Even over the last couple of years Diana has made great progress. When Bill first came, Diana couldn't make even a stab at his name. She called him "Jones Number Two" – after Gomer Jones who retired. Now she has a go at it. It's not an easy word, Hepplewhite. But she's almost there. You can see the difference.

'She used to be very depressed. Now, I think she has learned to live with frustration.'

Bill Hepplewhite trained as a remedial gymnast in the army, with the Medical Rehabilitation Unit in Chester. He set up his own medical rehabilitation unit in Singapore, then 'played soldiers for a while' before going to Chessington and finally leaving the army to come to Osborne. He never saw Diana at her most handicapped.

'Diana works in a group, but also as an individual. Actually so do most of the patients. I try to work with groups, but people's needs differ so much that often only individual work is practicable. Diana works at things like resisted exercises and so on. Even now she's continuing to make gains. She can straighten her right hand: she couldn't when I first came. Now she can use it more, for resting on something or pushing; she can raise it higher. Imagine . . . two years' work for her to raise her hand to her head.

'She *loves* the pool. She doesn't get any more movement there, but the water makes the exercises easier for her.

'It's not just the therapy though that makes Osborne matter so much to people like Diana. It's the environment that's damned important. Dressing for dinner, that sort of thing. The formality suits her. And we mostly get very active people here. Well-balanced. A lot between the ears.

'The atmosphere depends on who we have. Sometimes it can be dead, but whenever Diana comes she livens people up. She's a great organiser and a great participator. In the games she wins a lot of prizes – "once gentlemen's socks!"

'Osborne gives a great boost to morale. They tell each other how well they're doing. They may be lying, but they love it.'

Half-way through the morning comes a pause for hot drinks or milk, then – according to the individual programme – more exercises or possibly a visit to the occupational therapy unit, which is away from the main building and quite a walk for the less able.

Evelyn Penketh has been occupational therapist at Osborne for seven years. The unit is well-equipped, with facilities for painting, carpentry, enamelling, ceramics.

'Diana comes here occasionally to practise writing, but I don't see her often. She's a very positive personality. I remember once, she was here when I'd had some personal news which upset me, and she took over and set about getting a cup of tea and lit the gas stove for me. I remember that. It wasn't easy for her, with just one good hand, but she managed.'

At mid-day Diana invariably joins one of the small groups of patients making their way across the large croquet lawn beside the house and through the copse beyond to *Charlie's*, the golf club which is open to all Osborne residents.

Diana makes the most of this chance to recreate the kind of social life she enjoyed in the army and in her peacetime career. She meets old friends and makes new ones.

Gwynedd Laurie, ex-2nd Officer in the Wrens and a freewoman of the Saddlers Company, first met Diana at Osborne in 1971.

'It was my first time there. I was looking round to see whom I could join in the library before Diana, whom I had not previously met, seeing my plight, said, pointing to a vacant chair: "You! Here!" and I went and joined her group. She had very little speech at the time and I kept wanting to fill in the gaps for her. But Diana never let her lack of speech stop her in anything she wanted to do. She even tried to teach me billiard bowls, in which she's an Osborne champion player – without much success I'm afraid!'

Marianne Norris-Elye. 'I think some people feel that Osborne will be stuffed with brigadiers! And some are

petrified before they get here. That's why someone like
Diana can affect everyone else. Her influence is tremendous and inspiring. I've seen some of those who come
here, especially the men, creeping around and really miserable in themselves, and in a couple of days Diana's got
them going and they're different people. I think that
the idea that spouses should be admitted is good in some
ways, but should be tried out as an experiment before it's
permanently established. I think Diana would agree with
me that the stroke patients improve through their own
efforts – and need to leave off the constant attention of their
spouses!'

Rosemary Duncan. 'One of the things that's impressive
about Diana is that when she's here she's always got time
for other people. I remember once there was a man who'd
recently had a stroke and was very handicapped, and Diana
brought a shoe into the room where he was sitting and
demonstrated how to tie it up with one hand. And last
time I was here, there was some complication about my
husband coming, and I couldn't do the packing; Diana
insisted on doing it all herself with her one hand.

'She's an inspiration to others. A friend of mine had a
stroke seventeen years ago. It left her paralysed. Then she
recovered well physically, but she had virtually no speech,
only about five words. She saw a speech therapist privately
two years ago, but she had to give it up; she didn't feel she
was progressing and found the treatment expensive. I told
Diana about her, and Diana sent her leaflets. Now she goes
to a speech club, and she's taken on a completely new lease
of life. I don't know whether her speech is much improved
– I haven't seen her for a while – but she's quite different
in herself. I hear that she's had her hair done, she's bought
new clothes, she goes out with her husband.'

Back from the golf club to lunch; then after lunch a free afternoon. Some play golf, or croquet, or borrow a book from the handsome glass-fronted cases in the library. ('Patients are requested to play the game and not remove books without entering them in the ledger.') They can watch television in the special lounge, or settle down to the latest magazines in a comfortable country house-type living-room. Others prefer to seek peace and solitude on some bench tucked away in a corner of the gardens. Many, though, tired from the morning's exertions, are happy to sleep the afternoon away and meet again at tea.

However the afternoon has been spent, there's a general movement around 6.30 to gather in the library for a modest, pre-dinner get-together. Chits are signed for drinks chosen from a well-stocked bar; and conversation exchanged about the awfulness of the morning's exercises and the prospects for the morrow.

Everyone changes in the evening – nothing grandiose, but out of the trousers and sweat-shirts they've been wearing into something a little more formal; women are expected to wear dresses.

Dinner is the most formal meal of the day. On Fridays the governor attends; there's the Royal Toast and port is passed round. Even so, it's over quickly: perhaps under the influence of Queen Victoria, who expected meals to be over in thirty minutes flat!

Afterwards follows perhaps the most relaxed part of the day, as most of the visitors make up small groups to play competitive games. Diana is a dab hand at billiard bowls, played on a table with bulbous legs kicked by contesting officers over the years under the staring eyes of 'Dead Game' hanging on the wall.

Others go to the Games Room for dominoes, cards, shove ha'penny (a popular naval game) or Scrabble. ('Scrabble no good for me now,' explains Diana, it's the active games that she enjoys.)

Those who have cars (or spouses with cars) may take a short drive to a local pub, or simply sit and read until it's time for an evening cuppa and the chance of a last chat before bed.

Most are happy to retire early to their comfortable rooms, to sleep secure in the knowledge that a night nurse is available, until the Osborne clock (George III's, transported here from Kew), thoughtfully silenced during the night hours, chimes again with the morning tea.

One day succeeds another, uninterrupted except for the coming and going of visitors. The average stay is fourteen days. Many come only once; some stay only a week; others, like Diana, make repeated visits – for three weeks, or even four. As **Tony Chiverton** (who has been a porter here for twenty-four years) and his wife **Jean** say, 'Diana is always happy to get here, and there are tears when she goes.'

Jean Chiverton. 'But however upset she is, she manages. Even when she first came, and she was so depressed and cried a lot of the time, she didn't want anyone to help her. She could hardly move, but she insisted at meal times on fetching her own serviette and walking round the room until she found a spare place. The way she moved, that could take her ages. We can set aside convenient seats for the most handicapped, but she wouldn't have it. She'd move around at a snail's pace, on her own, until she found a hole. She has immense determination.'

Before they leave, all visitors have to visit the office on the lower ground floor to settle their accounts with Morriss Rumer, who handles all the administrative details.

Morriss Rumer was until recently the Steward of Osborne House, an executive officer of the Civil Service 'with a flair for money and people,' closely involved both with the State Rooms and the Convalescent Home.

'They're not all very pleased to have to come down here. Some of them would prefer to settle up upstairs and save themselves a little trip, but Diana's never like that. In fact she turns up quite often. Whenever I see her in the office, I say to her, "I know you're only here because you want something!" She'll be looking for paper, or envelopes, or sellotape, or paper clips. She's always busy with something. The first week here she can be quite a tartar. It's partly the drugs. Many of those here are very ill people. The drugs they have to take can make them react in ways they wouldn't normally. We understand that. The second week she's much calmer, more settled. We always enjoy having her. Whenever she's here she makes a difference to the spirit of the place.'

Clifford Woodcock, the chauffeur who drives the impressive black limousine which used to be the Queen Mother's, is another who remembers Diana as she was on her very first visits.

Clifford Woodcock. 'I've been driving here eight years, and seven years before that as relief. When I first saw her, she was in a dreadful state, really dreadful. You'd never have thought she'd make the progress she has. She could hardly speak. I could never understand a thing she said. I'd guess, I'd make wild guesses – nine times out of ten I was wrong, and it would upset her even more. But she's never given up. Some people do. You can see it. They make up their minds they're not going to improve. But she keeps on making progress. So appreciative, and very humorous. A lady of great character.'

There could hardly be a more striking contrast than between Clifford Woodcock's picture of Diana as she was and that of Diana today, as seen by Joan Crosley, coordinator of the four Isle of Wight speech therapists.

Joan Crosley came back to the Island in 1976 after working elsewhere for ten years, and is now a general practice therapist 'with a mixed bag:' a case-load of between sixty and seventy adults, treating perhaps twenty individuals each week, in addition to speech therapy care for about 160 pre-school children.

'Diana first contacted me in 1976 to ask me about the provision of speech therapy here and what was being done about speech clubs. I went to have tea with her at Osborne, and she gets in touch with me whenever she comes back to the Island. She always asks a lot of questions. She wants to know exactly what's going on.

'She approves of the way our speech clubs concentrate on therapy rather than the social side, though of course socialising is important; we recognise that it takes a special friend to listen and respond to a speech-handicapped person. At present we can have speech therapy at each session. We involve some nurses, health visitors, medical students, but at present no voluntary help.

'Since 1974 the service here has greatly improved, and speech therapy should now be available for anyone on the island. Some people get treatment twice a week: once, group therapy for two hours; once, individually for three quarters of an hour or so. The amount varies depending on age and need. People in the age-group thirty to fifty-five tend to get more, those over eighty-five less.

'Patients wanting to attend a speech club are mostly dependent on relatives and friends to bring them. We're all short of staff and time. The lay public mostly don't understand what's involved. That's what makes Diana's work so important.'

15　Milestones

During the years following the publication of Diana's letter, three events took place which not only gave her personal pleasure but – more important to her – marked stages of progress in her campaign for increased understanding of the problems of the speech-handicapped: the first special church service; the award of the Megan du Boisson prize; and the transmission of a play recounting Diana's experiences.

The most significant of these, for Diana, was undoubtedly the service, which was held for the first time in All Souls Church, Langham Place, in October, 1973. Diana described the prolonged preparations involved in the radio programme *You and Yours.*

The service is two years planning it and planning it and planning it. But I have done it now, and this service is going to be first in the British Isles, and I think annually in church.

Diana had the ready help of the then Rector of All Souls, John Stott.

John Stott has been connected with All Souls Church all his ordained life. After a brief period as curate, in 1950 he became Rector. In 1975 he became Rector Emeritus, and now spends three months every year travelling. Particularly interested in young people, he has led university missions here and abroad.

He is one of the Queen's chaplains and the author of many books.

'Diana comes of an Irish family with wide church connections. One of her cousins was Dr Gregg, Archbishop of Dublin, then of Armagh, Primate of All Ireland. She attended Sunday school regularly as a child.

'She and her mother used to attend Marylebone Parish Church until her mother moved to her present flat in 1941, when they began to attend All Souls or – after the church was bombed – St Peter's, Vere Street. They were fond of the previous Rector, Harold Earnshaw-Smith, and Mrs Law and Diana were very active in various church activities. I arrived in 1945, and have known them ever since.

'I find it extraordinary that Diana's Christian faith was never at any time disturbed by this terrible thing that happened to her. Her strong Christian belief throughout her life has been a support to her and an inspiration to others. Now that both Diana and her wonderful mother find it hard to attend services, I take them communion in their home several times a year.

'I was glad to help when Diana asked to see me about a possible service for the speech-handicapped. She had a three-fold concern clearly in mind. It was to assist and strengthen the people themselves and their relatives and friends; to inspire their medical helpers; and to awaken the general public to the difficulties. She felt that people were ready to be compassionate to the deaf and blind but not the dumb.'

The first service so obviously fulfilled a need that it has been repeated every year since. The pattern it follows is straightforward: ecumenical, with readings, a brief address, and prayers offered by members of the congregation of different convictions, some of them handicapped themselves. The tea party in the crypt afterwards gives everyone a chance to meet.'

Diana's support is both intuitive and practical. When on two occasions since, because of the reconstruction of All Souls, her service has had to be held elsewhere (at Marylebone and St Columba's), Diana played an active part in deciding their choice.

Michael Jackson. 'Her special service has always meant a great deal to her. She always plans an ecumenical service – with the Salvation Army playing their hymns, and Jews, Anglicans, Catholics all participating. We've had some ecumenical discussions – on vicars, choirs, bells and what not. She's very efficient and very practical. I remember one discussion on one church cut short when she leant forward and said firmly: *"No lavatories!"* So quite rightly that was out.'

Diana's capacity for organisation and publicity ensures that as many as possible hear of her service.* Copies of an advance notice sheet (the costs of which are borne by the Headley Trust set up by the Sainsbury family) are sent to the College of Speech Therapists to enclose in their monthly *Bulletin*, to local BBC stations throughout the country, and to any other associations – here and abroad – which might be interested. The BBC broadcast *Sunday* also always mentions it.

The average congregation is 500; others send cheques to help her cause. The service is not only an inspiration for the handicapped themselves but also fulfils Diana's urgent wish to make outsiders share in their situation, as **Gwynedd Laurie** describes.

'I found her service a very moving occasion. The church was packed. There was a young man with a speech defect

* See also page 182

who read the lesson, and he read it beautifully, without a single hesitation. I said to him afterwards, when we were all having tea and biscuits, "Weren't you nervous about it?" and he said, "No. When I was standing there I felt such a concentration of all the people listening, such a feeling that they were with me, that I knew it would be all right." The vicar who gave the address said that there were two people he always listened to, his wife because he had to, and Diana Law because he most *certainly* had to.'

The service means a great deal to Diana because of her own strong faith, though she is quite without dogmatism.

Always Church of Ireland. Now I like all denominations, all religions. Many people are struck down. I not resentful. Lots of people very bitter. But I'm not religious mad. Somebody is too much religion.

Before stroke always going to service at St Peter's. 8.30 pm. Lovely service. Hymns and praying. No sermon. Going to church difficult now because half-hour walk, hour and a half service, half hour walk, want to spend penny. Go on Sunday afternoon, very quiet. Pray, little talk with reception, or anyone.

Diana believes firmly that God intends her to make use of her own particular experiences for others. As she said on the radio programme, *In Town*, when asked if she felt she was achieving something for others she would not have done otherwise, she was in no doubt. 'I think God is willing me to do that to help other people.'

This same intention inspired the essay on her life since her stroke which she wrote with Joan Ellams and for which she was awarded the Megan du Boisson* prize. It was published in the DIG (Disablement Income Group) magazine.

* See also pages 44 and 95

Anne Handley-Derry. 'Diana received the money prize, but for one reason and another the presentation to her never took place. She was concerned about this, not for personal publicity – she's never wanted that – but because she hoped that press exposure would bring public recognition of the importance of her cause. That's what she's always worked for: for what it means to other people, not herself.'

Nonetheless, it was a distinction to be proud of; and only two years later the BBC broadcast of Alan Burgess's play perhaps conveyed to many more than ever before the awareness of what it must be like to have a stroke and be deprived of speech.

Make the Tongue Speak gives an imaginative account of Diana's experiences. Prunella Scales ('very nice') played the part of Diana, Jacqueline Morrell played herself; and Mrs Law wrote to Alan Burgess before casting to point out that 'I'm young: I mustn't have an old voice!'

This 40-minute play produced a great response. Many listeners wrote to Diana, and their opinions and their own experiences proved a source of mutual encouragement. Many made the point that the play had made them individually more determined to fight for a better existence and to make the most of their lives.

One writer summed up many others' views when she said: 'There's nothing like knowing you could have died for making you want to live. I know it can't be for ever, but it's very nice while it lasts.'

16   Speech at the Middlesex

In the mid-seventies Diana looked round to search for some way in which she could directly influence medical opinion and so help her cause. How better than to work through the hospital where she was already known and could communicate directly with those who would care for many of the stroke patients of the future: the Middlesex.

Catherine Taylor. 'As Diana improved, she used to drop in from time to time, just to keep me in touch. She'd bring me articles about herself or her speech clubs, pieces about her service, and so on. Then, in 1974, when I went into Nursing Administration, she asked if she could come in and speak to the student nurses. I went to the first talk she gave. It was inspiring. I'm sure that Diana gives many of the nurses a completely fresh insight into the problems of a patient who has had a stroke.'

Now Diana goes to the Middlesex not only to talk herself, but to act as a willing guinea-pig. The speech therapy department organises short courses not only for nurses in training but also for those who have the responsibility for what is described as 'maintenance work' – caring for stroke patients in various capacities after the initial crisis is over: nurses, district nurses, social workers, staff from old people's homes. The aim is to demonstrate, with the use of films and the co-operation of patients, what the effects of a stroke can be, what help is available, and what follow-up can be provided under expert direction by those without specialist skills. Diana regularly attends these, walking there on her own.

These sessions* often begin with a showing of the film made by the BBC for the Open Door of the Blackfriars Dysphasic Group (the group which, earlier, Diana might have attended instead of the CMRC). It was set up by a group of speech therapists with support from Guy's Hospital to provide the intensive speech therapy lacking in the National Health.

The wide range of people presented in this film demonstrates that dysphasia is not a problem for any one age group or type of person. From the young boy knocked off his bicycle at fifteen to the young woman left damaged as the result of a plastic surgery operation and the older man recovering from a stroke, they have all experienced similar problems to Diana's, and express the same needs and the same feelings.

They have difficulty in speaking to strangers. 'Worst thing . . . confusion. To make people understand.' The people they meet are embarrassed, or think they're mad or fools. 'In the pub, I go there, each person who is in moves away.' They won't wait while the dysphasic searches for words. 'People not patient.'

They all feel frustrated, from the older man who says, 'My speech, it's coming along fine, but I feel angry in *myself*,' to the young woman, a mother of two, who had a brain haemorrhage at twenty-four, who says with passion: 'My faculties are all there . . . but they swept me away . . . Takes a long time. People *butt* in, *butt* in. It makes me *mad*. Take the words out of my mouth. Want them to *wait* for me.'

---

* The lectures vary, but they share common ground; this account incorporates elements from more than one occasion.

They speak of the difficulty of finding jobs; the desire for re-training; the need to be accepted.

As a young man, formerly an architect and now operating a computer type-out, concludes: 'I just want the public to *forget* about us. No pointing – "He's got a limp!" So what!'

There is a general agreement that the progress they have made would be impossible without the speech therapy they are receiving. At the same time, a speech therapist describes the therapy available in the National Health as 'grudgingly provided,' and says that the work of the Blackfriars Group* is seriously threatened by lack of money: money needed to continue its work to help those affected, and to convince the general public that, in the words of one dysphasic, 'We have suffered from acute despair. But we are not cabbage-like people. We are just like you.'

DYSPHASIA AND COMPREHENSION

Next a speech therapist explains what causes dysphasia, and how to speak to dysphasics in order to be understood.

Doreen Cotter is Californian-born but has an English husband and did her speech therapy training in Britain. Originally a nursery school teacher, she trained at the Central School for Speech and Drama in London, in 'a unique atmosphere,' with its combination of voice and drama work. She taught at the North London College of Further Education before joining the Middlesex, and as part of her training carried out practical clinical work in California. She finds amenities better there, with places like Stanford particularly well endowed, but with no basic differences in techniques and standards.

'For spoken language to be understood, sound has to pass through the auditory channel to reach the language centre, where it is matched, interpreted and understood.

* See Appendix III

If there is an interruption at any stage, the message will not get through.

'There is only *one* language centre, in the dominant side of the brain; in 95 per cent of people this is on the left. It is not necessarily connected with left-handedness, although the 5 per cent of the population with the language centre in the right side includes a larger than average proportion of left-handers.

'When a stroke affects the dominant side the language centre is also damaged. In extreme cases, the language memory store will be totally obliterated; words become meaningless noises. Fortunately, this complete destruction is relatively rare.

'Intelligence is unaffected, and the memory of events and people is unchanged. Only the mechanism of speech, to convey and receive experience, is disrupted.

'This is an extremely frightening experience. These people know that once they could speak and understand, and now, suddenly, they no longer can. Some patients even believe they are going mad.

'It's important to realise that it's not the *hearing* which is affected. The patient will be bewildered and confused, and because he or she may fail to respond to even simple messages, it's not surprising that those who have never met this before, especially relatives, feel that he or she must be deaf, and start raising their voices.

'But this is not the difficulty. (Although, of course, the patient may have had hearing difficulties before, and in some cases the stroke may have also affected hearing.)

'The problem lies in the interpretation of the message. The words are heard, but mean nothing. For the patient, it's like listening to someone talking a foreign language which he speaks only imperfectly. Depending on the degree of impairment, he/she may pick up only the odd word here or there, or occasional phrases, or succeed in getting the gist of the conversation.

'For most patients, comprehension gradually improves, though it does not necessarily revert to normal.

'There are a number of ways in which those speaking to stroke patients can help both their comprehension and their confidence.

'First, obviously, don't shout. Speak in a normal voice, but take the trouble to be extra clear. Face the person you're talking to, because your expression will give him/her visual clues. Use gestures if you think they will help, but without being insultingly extravagant. Use short, simple language to start with, but never baby-talk. You're speaking to an adult, not a child. Keep your conversation specific; don't jump about from one topic to another. Especially, don't be in a hurry. It takes time for someone recovering from a stroke to comprehend a question, recall the words for an answer, and respond. If you haven't the patience to wait for a reply, you only discourage. And don't answer the question yourself! It's insulting to say, "How are you then? All right?" and rush off.

'Be prepared to make allowances. The patient will find it hard to concentrate for long. He/she will often be distracted: by noise, by other people, by things going on. Quiet and peaceful surroundings can help both of you to concentrate on the task of communication.

'Finally, remember that progress, though it may be steady over a long period, can in the short term seem very much like three steps forward two steps back. There is no regular pattern. Every individual presents a different picture. And every patient varies from week to week and day to day – almost from hour to hour. It's important not to get discouraged at apparent set-backs. These are normal. The effects of fatigue, drugs, depression, changes in medication or motivation – all these influence an individual's response.

'But, over a time, with care, treatment and stimulus, most patients' comprehension will improve, often very markedly.'

DYSPHASIA AND SPEECH RECOVERY

After explaining the difficulties of comprehension (input), the therapist goes on to describe the obstacles in the way of speech (output). Here Diana can contribute to the demonstration.

Joan Ellams. 'There are three different types of speech problems resulting from brain damage, whether through strokes, head injuries, Parkinson's disease, or multiple sclerosis. An individual may have one only, possibly a combination of two, or very rarely all three.

'The first is *dysarthria.* With this there is a malfunction of the muscles affecting breathing, voicing, and articulation; the message doesn't get through from the brain. The patient may also have trouble in swallowing, and drool because unable to control the saliva.

'Diana has never had dysarthria, but multiple stroke patients are very likely to suffer in this way. There are usually problems in intelligibility, and in very severe cases they may be able to say nothing, but only grunt. In less severe cases individuals may be difficult to understand because they speak much too fast or too slow. They may distort speech sounds, or substitute one sound for another – say "tup" for "cup." The quality of voice is affected: the pitch may be very low or very high.

'To be able to speak a patient must have control over the muscles affecting breathing; the larynx; those moving the tongue, mouth, soft palate and so on; so we start by exercising these.

'First, you can encourage the patient to produce simple vowel sounds – ah, ee, oo, etc. Then simple breathing exercises: breathing in to a count of 1,2,3, and then out to 1,2,3; then progressing to 4,5,6, and so on. What matters is the deliberate control of the breathing.

'Then go on to simple lip and tongue exercises, and the reproduction of all the basic sounds in the language:

p,b,t,th,s, and so on. The patient can then go on to put these together with a simple vowel sound, either before it or after it or in between: pa, ap, appa.

'They move on to simple consonant combinations: star stay, store; play, please, plate, etc.

'If the patient's dysarthria is less severe, you can move on to a more demanding stage. Get him or her to read a passage, then work on the *way* it's read – speeding it up or slowing it down as necessary. Finally you can help the patient practise stress and intonation, to express the difference, for example, between "*Tom* went to Brighton," and "Tom went to *Brighton.*"

'This is only the very last stage. The first stages are very important. If a patient is untreated he or she becomes depressed, isolated and unmotivated. The treatment is *psychologically* helpful, quite apart from other benefits. What matters to patients isn't *how* they communicate, but that they manage to in some way, whatever that way may be.

'The second speech disorder is *dysphasia*, generally caused by a lesion in the dominant side of the brain and affecting all aspects of language function. This is how her stroke affected Diana.

'With expressive dysphasia the patient knows what he or she wants to say, but can't find the words. The frustration is enormous. We can feel a taste of what it's like when we can't recall a name; we know it's on the tip of our tongue, but we can't recapture it. That, intensified, is how it is for dysphasics all the time.

'They have difficulty in finding individual words, then difficulty in putting those words together in a phrase. They may also suffer from perseveration (continuing to use one word for others) and paraphasia (the confusion of one word or sound with another).

'Diana, as you know, has made immense progress from her early stages, but she can demonstrate the problems she still faces and give you some idea of how to go about recalling speech in your patients. Remember that what you are helping the patient to do is *not* to learn each individual word, but to *practise the technique of recall.* You can use tape-recorders, video-machines and so on, but a paper and pencil and straightforward material cut from magazines are just as effective.

'One of the techniques that Diana still uses is automatic speech.

'Diana, what number comes after 8?'

(Counting): '*1,2,3,4,5,6,7,8,* nine.'

'What day comes after Wednesday?'

'*Sunday, Monday, Tuesday, Wednesday,* Thursday.'

'And what month comes after July?'

(Much slower and with hesitation): '*January, February, March, April . . . June . . .*' (She stops.)

'Yes, Diana finds that harder. Numbers she always manages. You may find patients much happier with words than numbers, or the other way round. You can try other sequences as well, depending on your patients' interests. Familiar songs are often successful.

'A very useful word-recaller is to use pictures.

'Diana, what's in this picture? And this? And this?'

(Diana correctly identifies each in turn, sometimes immediately, sometimes after a pause. Occasionally she fixes on a detail in the picture rather than the whole. If the pause gets too long, she starts to draw out the initial letter of the word on the table with her finger, repeating the action until she manages to capture the word.)

'Another cue is to ask the patient to complete a sentence.

'There is someone knocking at the –'

'*Door.*'

'Please pass the salt and –'

'*Pepper.*'

'Diana finds that easy. It's harder to answer simple questions.

'What do we do with soap?'

'Wash.'
'What do we do with scissors?'
'Cut.'
'What do we wear on our feet?'
'Socks.'
'What else?'
'Shoes.'
'What else?'
'Mmmm . . . slippers.'

'It's more difficult still for patients to formulate a whole sentence. You suggest a word as a stimulus. They have to understand it, select the right words for the response, put them together, and say them before they slip away again.

'Diana, say a sentence using the word *coat*.'
'I have a new coat.'
'Want.'
'I want a cup of tea.'
'Pink.'
'What pink? Colour pink? Yes? The dress is pink.'

'Then you can ask patients to describe what they see in pictures. As you've seen, Diana does this well. Much harder for her is to define a word.

'Diana, what is a bridge?'

(Diana indicates with her hand what a bridge is, but struggles with only partial success to put the concept together.)

'You see, even Diana finds this a problem. Again, the point to remember is the importance of communication. As long as the patient is progressing in understanding and communicating, coming across various stumbling-blocks like definitions don't matter.

'A more complex exercise you can try with those whose understanding and speech has already improved is to read a short story, or even just a paragraph of a few sentences, and ask the patient to retell it to you as completely as possible. Obviously, this should only be attempted in the later stages.

F

'The third speech disorder is *dyspraxia*. This is a disorder in articulation. The patient is *capable* of muscle movement, but doesn't know how to make the correct muscle movements, or makes them inconsistently. There is difficulty in getting certain sounds, especially the beginning sounds of words. Diana still has some dyspraxia.

'The exercise here is to get the patient to work alongside you in front of a mirror. Practise simple repetitive speech – vowel sounds, consonants, simple sound combinations, simple words, simple sentences – so that the patient can study and copy the movements made in the mirror.

'Follow this with repetitive speech on its own, then reading aloud, then structured conversation situations in much the same way you've already heard with Diana.

'I would like to emphasise again that you are dealing with adults. Remember that even though they may not be able to speak, they may understand very well. Don't talk over their heads, or discuss their cases in front of them.

'Try to make sure they understand what has happened to them; reassure them that they're not stupid or mad. Do your best to set aside a regular time each day to talk to each individually.

'It helps if the environment is kept quiet. Patients find it hard to concentrate, and are easily distracted by noise and bustle. Relax. Talk reasonably slowly, and keep what you say short.

'Start with simple things. Don't try to stretch patients too soon. Let them succeed. If they have difficulties, don't press them too hard – help them with the missing word, or leave it for another time.

'Involve them in activities as much as you can. Don't avoid talking to them: on the contrary, encourage them to speak.

'Above all, take your time. It's not easy when you're rushed to wait and wait for an answer which never seems to come, but this is what's needed. And, if you're in touch with relatives, remind them tactfully of all these points.'

DYSLEXIA AND DYSGRAPHIA

Finally, the therapist discusses the difficulties of reading and writing.

Doreen Cotter. 'Reading, writing and speech are the same, in that they are all means of communication, but through different channels, one visual, one aural. To read and write, a patient needs both vision (acuity and visual field) and the ability to move a pen.

'Some stroke patients, in addition to sight defects they have already had before their stroke, suffer from hononymous hemianopia, which cuts off the field of vision, usually on one side. This means that they lose one part – for example the right-hand side – of the visual field of each eye. This increases difficulties of reading and writing, in that letters and words will disappear as these move out of the visual field.

'Many stroke patients also have basic manipulative problems. If, as frequently happens, their stroke damages that part of the brain which controls the dominant side, it affects the hand that normally writes, so that apart from everything else they have great difficulty in actually putting the letters on the paper – either by trying to use a paralysed hand or having to transfer to the hitherto weaker side.

'After establishing any physical difficulties involved – that is, visual or mechanical complications – a speech therapist will start to test the patient with the aim at establishing the level at which he or she will just succeed. This will probably involve simple tests like matching words and pictures; reading simple sentences; following simple written commands.

'A patient may have very elementary difficulties in perceiving letters and shapes. Beyond this, he/she may understand letters but be unable to connect them into sentences. It's not only the ability to perceive, but to retain the perception long enough to do something with it.'

Joan Ellams now demonstrates writing techniques with the help of Diana.

'To help the patient, different techniques are possible, depending on the level of breakdown.

'First and simplest is *tracing* written letters, then progressing to *copying*; there can be an intermediate stage, following a sequence of dots, as we used to do when we were children. I would suggest, first, letters using only horizontal and vertical lines: I,H,E. Then those also using diagonals: M,N,W. Then those with curves: P,B,S.

'Next you can move on to words, then from words to phrases. Progress may be slow, and uncertain. Diana can now copy well, as she will show us, but she has little spontaneous writing.'

Diana successfully copies down, in a felt-tipped pen, *CHILD, child, the child is playing.* She then goes on to fill in missing words: I was tired so I went to *bed*; I went to the *Midd Hosp*. Next she adds missing letters: FIS*H*, TABL*E*, *C*OMB. (P-PER is temporarily baffling: Diana tries, but doubtfully, P*E*PER, and eventually after some thought successfully gets P*A*PER.) Then she tackles simple anagrams. BDE she rapidly reassembles as BED. TAIRN takes several painstaking tries (and some help) before she manages to put together TRAIN.

Numbers offer no difficulty. Diana spontaneously writes 1 to 10 without a prompt.

Real problems emerge when she is asked to write down complete phrases. She puzzles for some time over 'a cup of tea,' and after a long pause writes *cup* well over on the right edge of the page. When Joan Ellams explains that she has left no room for 'of tea', Diana first expostulates, then laughs at her mistake.

'Some therapists like to concentrate on lower case letters, but for many patients upper case are easier to form. The main thing is to progress in stages – first letters, then words, then sentences. With some patients you can start phonic work earlier than with others: B says "b", P says "p", and so on. It all depends on the individual. Treatment must be flexible.

'One small practical hint. If you clip a sheet of paper to a board, and clip or stick a sponge back on to the board, your patient will be able to write on it with one hand without having it slip all over the place.

'Try not to use childish material – ABCs and so on. Use words cut from newspapers instead; again, because you're dealing with adults, not children. There's a great lack of adequate printed work to use with dysphasics.

'Encourage your patients to make their own vocabularies, like Diana. She has three – set out in ordinary address books: one is a shopping list, one a straight-forward dictionary, and one a letter-writing book, with names and addresses and conventional phrases. She may not be able to *recall* a word, but she knows where it is in her vocabulary, she can look it up, and copy it down; it's not spontaneous, but in this way she can communicate through writing. Dictionaries for young readers can also be helpful.

'Again, you must remember the needs of the individual. Men of the older generation may have written very little even before their stroke – it was their wives who wrote any letters which were necessary. If you can help them to read the newspaper headlines and the TV programmes, this may be as much as they did before and as much as they need now.

'There should be specialist help for you to call on, even if only sporadically.

'Every area now has a speech therapist responsible for everyone in that area needing speech therapy. There should be a regular link between the local speech therapist and day care centres. It may not be possible to have regular visits, but the occasional one-off visit should be quite on the cards. Speech therapists are happy to offer their services around. If you need a speech therapist to guide your efforts, then ask and *keep on asking.*'

Diana is delighted to be able to help with these sessions. She is proud of the Middlesex and what it already does for speech therapy; she wants to see the same approach repeated throughout the country.

'My hospital the best! Others hospitals must be good too.'

17 M.B.E.

In the New Year Honours List of 1978 Diana was awarded the MBE.

Anne Handley-Derry. 'It meant a lot to Mrs Law when Diana got her MBE. More than to Diana herself, perhaps; but she was glad to have it, not personally, but because she hoped it would draw attention to the needs of her cause.'

Letter written two months before announcement. Keep it dark. Mother told and Joan Ellams, also Anne Handley-Derry and Leo. Otherwise nobody knew about it. I asked my mother to come too, and Joan Ellams to represent the speech therapy profession.

Major-General Peter Gillitt (I knew him before the war and in Berlin) met me at the Palace. I saw the whole thing. Me, one man in wheelchair and one crippled man very near by, in stands with relatives. Equerries help men. I walk alone.

A long wait. Very long way to the ballroom. The Queen speaks to me, but I forget what. A hundred and fifty decorations and honours. Tired out, the Queen. Sometimes sword, sometimes not. Then very long way away to the passage. Then an interview with journalists, then photographs, then with my mother and Joan Ellams to Leo and Anne Handley-Derry for lunch.

Mary Law. 'It was on the 21st February at half past ten that Diana was to be at the Palace to receive the MBE at the hands of Her Majesty the Queen. We got up early and we got dressed and we were ready to start at ten minutes to ten. Miss Ellams arrived, the car arrived . . . We entered the main gate and we went to the side door, because my daughter had to use the lift. . . . We were greeted by a general covered with ribbons and gold lace and things, and the minute he saw my daughter he said "Ah, Diana!" and shook her by the hand. Then my daughter went her way and Miss Ellams and I went ours . . . to the ballroom, where we sat one-third of the way down on the outside of the aisle, where we had a good view of all that was going on.

'We had music, piano music and orchestral music, not too loud, and people kept coming in, and eventually the Beef-eaters arrived and then the Gurkhas, so we knew that the next person to come would be Her Majesty, and there she was, looking as usual very charming. Then it was mostly the men who came in. There weren't very many women.

'So in due course Diana arrived. She stood in front of the Queen, and she made her little bob and took three steps forward. The Queen spoke to her, and said she'd heard how well she'd done. She didn't attempt to shake hands, because evidently she'd been told that Diana's right hand was paralysed. And then she went off. There were very few people after her.

'And then we duly went through all the corridors, past the beautiful pictures which we hadn't time to look at, and past various marble children lying stretched on tables. . . . Then we were photographed in various positions.

'Then to a lunch party. We had a very pleasant lunch and we left about three o'clock and came home. I went to sleep. Miss Ellams sat and contemplated. As for Diana – she never told me what *she* did, but I imagine she wandered about!

'At six o'clock we had the beginnings of the party when people began to arrive. We didn't have any grand drink and things. We just had vin rosé, and the very nicest mixture of biscuits Marks and Spencers could provide.

'And we looked back and thought what a happy day we'd had, and how kind everyone had been. Rosamond Day who had provided the glasses and couldn't have been more helpful, and Ann and Leo Handley-Derry who gave the lunch party and arranged everything so well. . . .

'There hadn't been a shadow of any sort. Even though the day had been so dull and dreary we hadn't noticed it.'

18 Miracle on a shoestring

The award of her MBE served only to spur Diana on to greater efforts. Her belief in the size of the problem the speech-handicapped faced was confirmed when, after the publication of an article on her experiences in the January 1978 edition of *Good Housekeeping*, she received a further two hundred letters describing similar difficulties.

Further publicity brought yet more letters. She spoke on many radio programmes: *World at One, You and Yours, Woman's Hour, PM, In Town, Does He Take Sugar?* and on television in *Lost for Words*; also on many local radio stations. Many more articles appeared: in *the remedial therapist, Nursing Times, MIMS Magazine (for GP's)*, the *Society of Friends* newsletter, and again many local papers.

The response helped to keep her going.

Thanks to her scribes, and her own efficient filing system, she kept up a high-pressure correspondence with her various contacts: people like Alfred Morris, Sir Sigmund Sternberg, Lady Masham, Patrick Jenkin, Lady Jeger, Jack Ashley, Lord Seebohm, Lord Longford, Lynda Chalker; doctors, nurses, the Disablement Income Group, and many, many others; chalking up some successes along the way, pressing on always towards the next issue.

In mid-1978 she succeeded in having questions answered in Parliament on two occasions.

On July 20th 1978 Robin Hodgson (her cousin) asked

a whole series of questions on the provision of speech therapy, covering aspects of training, demand, the lack of available figures on adults requiring it: statistics obtained included comparative figures for the provision of speech therapists by the different Health Authorities at September 1976.

In a written answer to Lena Jeger's question (July 7th 1978), Roland Moyle reported: 'Good progress has been made in moving towards the 20-year target for Great Britain of 2,500 speech therapists (whole-time equivalent) recommended in the 1972 Quirk Report on Speech Therapy Services. Numbers have grown from about 800 in 1972 to about 1,430 in 1976 (the latest available figure), but we are still some way from being able to meet all the needs of patients. The development of speech therapy as with all other aspects of rehabilitation remains a priority area for development.'

Peggy Dalton adds a personal viewpoint.

'I entirely support Diana's campaign for more speech therapists and better use made of them. It would be a help if a more flexible attitude were adopted towards grants. Graduates in particular tend to come off badly. Many of them have to scrape financially and do the course in two years instead of three. Although this may not always matter academically – they may have exemptions, for example, because they have already qualified in psychology – they do miss a whole year of observation and treatment. They cope, but it's not ideal.

'Pay is better since the Quirk report. When I first qualified I was getting £800 pa! And on the whole, trained therapists can rely on finding the kind of work they want, although if they are set on working only in the London area there may be less choice of jobs.

'I think it will be an improvement when therapists can

train for four years instead of three, since I think after one or two years in general practice a therapist really needs to specialise. The field is too big for one person to be able to keep up with developments in all areas. As it is, therapists here tend to remain isolated from experience in other countries. There isn't the money available for travel abroad, and reading papers is no substitute for personal observation.

'Not that it's easy even to keep up with published papers. I can just about cope with those published in the English-language press, but there may be valuable research carried out in Germany or France that I never hear about because of the language barrier.'

TOWARDS MORE SPEECH CLUBS

As month after month went by, more and more speech clubs were started; and thrived. By the end of 1979, seven years after Diana's initial letter, 209 clubs had been founded – thirty-two of them by the WRVS. The movement had also spread abroad, with clubs started in Australia and New Zealand by therapists who had visited groups here and subsequently written to Diana.

Many of these owe their existence directly to Diana's vision and encouragement.

Michael Jackson. 'Her speech clubs are her guiding light. She's thrown all her energies and experience into promoting them. She uses her contacts and her position into organising others to get things done. And it works.'

Although so many clubs have already been started, far more are still needed. There are areas of the country where the nearest one might still be a very long journey away. Often the need is simply not recognised.

Barbara Deason. 'It's not surprising that social workers and doctors in general simply don't realise the size of this problem. At a recent conference a doctor said that the average GP may see only one speech-handicapped adult a year, and each social worker may have only one speech-handicapped client. It's only when you put all these separate ones together that you realise the numbers involved.

'I've recently tried to set up speech clubs in an area where there has never been one before. The Education Authority agreed to pay, but the local speech therapist said there was no need for a club offering therapy. We now have a stroke club which organises all sorts of social activities. This obviously fulfils a need too – people come to it readily – but I can't help wondering if they might not possibly want more. I feel that if a speech club were actually started, the same need might be uncovered as it was when we first opened up in Camden.'

Diana remains deeply concerned that the standards of these clubs should be maintained. Since she knows so well what speech therapy has done for her, she insists that a trained speech therapist must be available at each session of each speech club. She sees the risk that, otherwise, play will take over from work and no real progress towards speech be achieved.

Volunteers nevertheless have a vital part to play.

Joan Ellams. 'Personally, I'm all in favour of all sorts of group therapy. Therapeutic, social, all have their uses. I'm in favour of volunteers – though some speech therapists aren't. I want to see everything. All systems go.

'Ideally, volunteers should have professional guidance, but it doesn't always work like that. Even so, a group gives confidence, and an opportunity for practice. It's less spoon-fed, but still sheltered. It gives support. And it's particularly valuable when patients start to progress – in later stages – more through the course of time than through direct therapy.'

Michael Jackson. 'Volunteers can certainly have a most valuable part role. For example, Valerie Eaton Griffith's book, *A Stroke in the Family*, shows how friends and neighbours can co-operate to help a stroke victim. It's a helpful and a genuinely humble book, by someone who saw something to be done and simply went ahead and did it in the best way she could. It's a book we recommend our students to read, especially for the light it shows on the relationships between people. Another reason is that it's the kind of book that patients' relatives will read and then mention to the speech therapist. However, we always emphasise that the book is not, and was not intended to be, a treatise on aphasia; not all patients should be expected to do as well as Patricia Neal.'

Dr A-M T. 'Obviously, it would be marvellous if everyone could have all the professional speech therapy they need, but it's not going to be possible in the foreseeable future. We mustn't overlook the fact that in the middle of Yorkshire people needing help with their speech disabilities will almost certainly have volunteers or no one.

'I'm sure too that Diana would be the first to agree that quite apart from the speech therapy volunteers have an enormous part to play. They break the isolation. This is almost the most important thing they can do. They visit. They encourage neighbours to come. They maintain a social contact with the outside world. They don't need special skills. If they have understanding and sympathy, they can contribute greatly to a patient's efforts at recovery.'

TOWARDS GREATER UNDERSTANDING

Diana continues her work to gain far greater official understanding of speech handicap as the disablement it is.

She is particularly alert for occasions when references to the 'handicapped' appear to exclude the speech-handicapped. A typical example occurred when the Manpower Services Commission advertised their *Fit for Work* award, offering prizes to firms with the most constructive policy for the employment of the disabled, without specifically including the speech-handicapped; Diana wrote to the Chairman to point out this discrepancy.

When Alfred Morris's paper on the problems of the disabled did likewise, Diana wrote to him too. She also wrote one of her own letters to one of her contacts at the DHSS:

20.6.78.

Dear Mr Perry
1) How are you?
2) *The Times* = 14.6.78 Alfred Morris
3) Blind & deaf = OK?
   Speech disorders = NO
4) I furious!!!
                    Yours ever
                    Diana Law

Every time the blind and deaf are mentioned in prayers on the BBC – but not the speech-handicapped – she gets in touch with BBC Religious Broadcasting. 'I ring up and scold them!'

Diana feels that the needs of the speech-handicapped are often ignored, even by those who are closely involved in helping the disabled: a recent advertisement for NAIDEX*, while mentioning many other specific disabilities, has no reference to those with speech handicaps.

She believes that the public (and often the medical pro-

* National Aids for the Disabled Exhibition

fession too) have no concept of the problems created by the lack of adequate speech. She is determined to enlighten them.

In pursuit of this goal, Diana became increasingly concerned about certain aspects of the policy of the Department of Health and Social Security towards those handicapped by speech disabilities. With the help of Joan Ellams, a meeting was arranged with officials of the DHSS at Hannibal House, the Elephant and Castle, in mid-November 1978.

Here Diana and Joan Ellams raised various points; specifically, the need for improved statistics on those requiring speech therapy, more research, and better facilities.

One aspect which Diana felt was particularly important was the lack of any direct reference to speech-impaired people in the Chronically Sick and Disabled Persons Act, and that this reflected a general lack of knowledge of and interest in this particular handicap. As she later wrote (through a scribe) to emphasise, 'It is unfortunate that the word "dumb" is used (in the National Assistance Act 1948) as this does not really describe the condition of most people with a speech handicap.

'As speech handicap is different from either physical or mental handicap I do think it should be given particular reference. Very few people, even within the DHSS itself, are aware of speech handicap and its nature, and there are occasions when speech-handicapped people have had great difficulty in securing social service facilities relating in particular to financial situations simply on the basis of their speech handicap.'

Betty Byers Brown, adviser on speech to the DHSS, later took up this point and emphasised that the DHSS now 'does in fact recognise that speech handicap is a particular category of disability . . . I think it is probably a matter of continuing education of Departments and the public. . . . The Act as now drafted carries the necessary inference if people interpret it properly. We are naturally concerned that individual speech-handicapped persons and their relatives realise this and that is where your publicity is effective.'

As part of her function as Adviser, Betty Byers Brown also emphasised to Diana that she tried 'to increase awareness of the pervasive nature of speech handicap in many ways. I draw official attention to all the new trends in therapy and to any neglected group. I try to get money for research and development e.g. for post-stroke rehabilitation. I see that DHSS staff are invited to meetings of Area Speech Therapists or to Conferences. I accompany DHSS staff to centres where treatment for speech-handicapped people is carried out or is contemplated and explain the nature of the conditions. . . .'

Ironically, the circumstances of this meeting at the Elephant and Castle were such that they seemed to Diana to symbolise society's capacity to overlook the needs of the disabled. Representatives of the DHSS did their best to ensure a suitable welcome for her, but this nonetheless involved an entrance through a dirty basement, a climb up seven steps with no handrail, and an awkward trip in a defective wheelchair. Rapid letters were sent off in all directions; not for her own sake, but for all those handicapped people who are in this way automatically relegated to the rank of second-class citizens.

PENSION PROBLEMS
In the same spirit, when complications ensued in 1979 over the payment of her retirement pension, Diana joined battle again; not only for herself but, she hoped, for all those in similar circumstances.

In February 1979 Diana received a routine form from the North Fylde Central Offices at Blackpool of the Department of Health and Social Security enclosing a routine letter and leaflet concerning her retirement pension which would become due on her sixtieth birthday in June 1979.

Although the leaflet describing the factors affecting pensions stated that those already in receipt of an invalidity pension would receive an augmented retirement pension, the attached form seeking information to enable the final pension to be calculated did not appear to include any suitable space for details of invalidity pensions.

Diana sought advice from five competent advisers, who all found themselves baffled; and, unwilling to make mistakes through filling it in wrongly, wrote, through a scribe, for clarification to the DHSS offices at Colquoun House in Broadwick Street. In April she received a further letter from the Blackpool Offices asking for the form and offering help. She wrote back immediately explaining the circumstances, enclosing the filled-in form and asking for it to be returned if it was incorrect.

For the next few months there followed a protracted correspondence, complicated initially by the unavailability – because of the postal strike in Eire – of a copy of Diana's birth certificate.

However, at the beginning of June, shortly before her birthday, Diana received notice from the Aldershot office of the DHSS that, while waiting to hear from the Pension Office the amount of Retirement Pension to which she would be entitled, they would stop paying invalidity benefit the day before her birthday. Meanwhile, 'You should claim Supplementary Benefit at your local office.'

Diana wrote to point out that due to her disablement she would have great difficulty in applying in person for Supplementary Benefit, and asking whether it would not be possible to send her instead a cheque or giro.

After this letter followed letter, on Diana's part, without response and without money. An excerpt from one she wrote – again through her scribe – to the DHSS (Supplementary Section) at Tavistock Square on June 28th gives a vivid picture of her increasing desperation.

'. . . As I received no reply to my letter of 15 June I

then wrote to Blackpool on 21 June and also to Regency St. Again on 21 June. Having once again received no reply, I wrote again on 26 June to Blackpool and also to Regency St.

'I am getting so desperate for help that I rang Blackpool in the morning of 27 June (it has cost me a lot of money) where I was told by a woman that my papers had gone to Edinburgh. The person at Blackpool was very helpful and said she would phone Regency Street and get them to ring me and do something about my problem.

'As I had no reply by 2.30 that day I then went to Gt Portland Street PO. I went there and was told all sorts of excuses but I sat down and refused to go until I had spoken to someone in authority, people were very good to me and I eventually spoke to the Head Postmaster who very kindly rang Blackpool, Aldershot, Regency Street, who told him that Tavistock Square WC1 was the correct office. The Head Postmaster at Gt Portland Street then filled in a form for me and I signed it. I was there one and a half hours. I am writing this letter to ask *what* you intend to do and how long you expect me to wait before I get my pension which is long overdue.'

Further letters followed to various suggested offices, culminating, on July 23rd, in one interim payment of £19.50. It was not until August 9th that Diana finally received from the Regency Street branch a girocheque to cover the back payments from 14.6.79, after the date when her invalidity pension had been stopped.

During all this period Diana was under great pressure and short of money, confused by the number of offices involved, and worried by letters which remained unanswered.

My pension stop on June 8th. Then no more money. All those weeks. What about other people? What do they do?

Me, I write letters, and look at the time it takes! What about people who don't write letters? How long do they wait? Some handicapped people, their families perhaps not very good at fighting. Why do we have to fight like this? We need a better way.

'MY CLUB' AND THE CICELY NORTHCOTE TRUST

It was fortunate that during the time of all this increasing pressure, some extra help – other than that of Diana's devoted friends and scribes – gradually became available.

After the publication of the *Daily Telegraph* letter Diana and her friends had founded an association, known at first simply as the Association of Speech Clubs, to keep the initial impetus going and to provide enquirers with some help and information. The original secretary and treasurer died, and Diana and her friends – Anne Handley-Derry, Tom Newton, Barbara Deason and Joan Ellams – found it increasingly difficult to keep up with the demands of the association and the subsequent correspondence.

In 1979 they began to rethink its needs and aims. It was at just this time that the Cicely Northcote Trust in Lambeth came forward with a proposition.

Janet Wells, administrator of the Cicely Northcote Trust, took a degree in Social Administration at Nottingham University, but subsequently found herself teaching in comprehensive and secondary modern schools, often in urban areas with many social problems. She travelled extensively here and abroad, and on returning to the UK applied for the post at the Trust because this would enable her to live and work in the same area.

'I read about Diana for the first time in about 1975 or 1976, and felt that her cause was one which the Cicely Northcote Trust might be able to help.'

'The Trust was started in 1909 by Hugh Northcote in memory of his sister who had died of paratyphoid at only eighteen. He was inspired by a visit to Boston, USA, where he found social work backing up medical work in a way at that time less developed here. Originally the Trust was closely connected with St Thomas's Hospital, and began by employing almoners (social workers) who could help to ameliorate the home conditions of medical patients.

'After the start of the National Health Service the almoners became part of it, so the Trust money was no longer needed for this purpose. We still have links with the hospital, and we remain closely connected with the district, but our interests are not limited by geographical or institutional considerations.

'Ideally, what the Trust aims to do is to fund groups for a period to enable them to become self-supporting, so that other groups in turn may be taken on. We've helped to fund occupational therapy units, hostels for VD clinics, children's play facilities, supportive groups of all kinds, youth and senior clubs.

'From hearing of Diana I believed that her cause was clearly of importance to a lot of people and one which needed all the support it could get.

'To start with, I thought we might be able to start a speech club in this building. Then, when the solicitors here moved out, I thought of offering the space to her for use as an office. I knew she was working from a small bedroom, and I felt that a charity which aims to be a national force must need more room. She would also have the backing of an established charity, which could offer her further contacts through the Health Service and the Hospital. We had received a grant from the General Charitable Trust of Mr Maurice B.Reckitt; and partly because he had suffered from a mild stroke himself and would be sympathetic to the cause of the speech-handicapped, and partly because the Committee of Management of the Cicely Northcote Trust sympathised with the self-help aspect of Diana's work, it was suggested that we should back her and support her until an independent association could be set up.

'Diana came and met the Council, and impressed them all with her personality and courage. She was persuaded that there was much she could do with the help of the Trust that she would find difficult without. We offered her an office here virtually rent-free, my help and time, and the use of volunteers.

'Since then some of the practicalities have proved difficult. It's quite a journey for Diana from the West End to Lambeth. Understandably, she has been reluctant to transfer any of her files. One can understand this, just as one can understand her impatience: she is aware of people suffering, she wants things done immediately, now.

'We need a co-ordinating person to see that more work gets done faster. One of the questions we're considering at the moment is whether to spread what money we have thinly over a longer period, or to make use of it in a shorter more intense involvement.

'Even so, in the past year we have made progress. I've convened meetings, and done a lot of behind-the-scenes clerical work. I've done hours of typing, duplicating and collating. It's very time-consuming work, but again we've no staff to help. We've done a lot of the back-up work for Diana's church service. And the Trust, through my efforts and those of volunteers, have produced a duplicated version of the Register of Speech Clubs from information collected by Diana*.

'We have also most recently helped with the establishment of a Steering Committee to found an independent charity for dysphasic adults* to carry on Diana's work. The Steering Committee has drawn up the Constitution which sets out the objects of the proposed association: briefly, "to promote and provide, or assist in promoting and providing, facilities for the rehabilitation of adults suffering from speech and language disorders following brain damage

* See Appendix II

and to act in any manner which now is or hereafter may be deemed by law to be charitable."

'We hope that we have in this way helped with some of the spadework necessary for the expansion of Diana's project, and that this Steering Committee will become the nucleus of the new charity.

'The association itself is now in a period of transition between the work of one person in a bedroom to the organisation of a national charity. Diana is its guiding light. There are things she can do that no one else can. There is no point in her wasting herself in duplicating what others are doing. Diana is needed above all for the publicity she brings to her cause, and the people she contacts. Let someone else write the routine letters, and free her for the work only she can do.'

Barbara Deason. 'Diana asked me to be one of those co-opted on to the committee of her Association of Speech Clubs, which then turned into the current Steering Committee.

'Diana feels that progress has been slow, but in my experience setting up groups like this – and I've been concerned with quite a number – always takes time. Establishing the constitution has taken a lot of discussion, but it's no use trying to rush this. If there are ambiguities or gaps, a lot of trouble can be caused later to those trying to abide by it. It takes a long time too for those concerned to get used to it, to get to know all that they ought to know. Diana knows already – it's in her bones – but others don't. They must become really deeply involved: otherwise they start to drop out.

'We have to plan now for the future. This takes thought and dedication. And everything has to be done in our free time. We meet once a month very regularly. It takes me $1\frac{1}{2}$ hours travelling time, plus the actual meeting and any preliminary work or follow-up that needs doing. It takes quite a chunk out of my month. If it took any longer I couldn't do it. I would feel guilty about the time taken from my own work.

'Without the help of the Northcote Trust we could never have got so far. Janet Wells has given us a lot of assistance, and their typing and duplicating facilities have enabled us to do the work which would otherwise never have been done. We would be where we were a year ago. We have definitely made progress.

'I often say Diana wants everything done yesterday! But without her prodding us we would never get through half what we do.

'What we have to concentrate on now is good organisation, a central place, and a good co-ordinator, so that Diana will be free to concentrate on publicity. I'm sure Diana in her business life must have delegated like mad, and that's the stage we've got to now.

'And she certainly hasn't lost any of her commercial acumen. I've recently started selling things in Camden Lock, and Diana asked what profit I expected to realise on my stock, and when I said 10 per cent she said, "No, my dear, you must take 20 per cent at least!" '

Anne Handley-Derry. 'What we need now above all is the money to pay a good co-ordinator so that Diana can be freed from so much of her routine work. The association needs her at its head for her drive and understanding and inspiration. If she were free to concentrate on the publicity she's so good at, we could expand and achieve much more.

'So far Diana's performed a miracle on a shoestring. But before we can go on to even greater achievements an administrative office must be established with settled finances.'

VOCAL

Diana spoke for her Association at the first ever day conference held by VOCAL in October 1979 at the Middlesex Hospital.

Yvonne Edels. 'VOCAL was established back in 1977 at the College of Speech Therapists, who wanted to co-ordinate the activities of charities concerned with speech handicaps. It's proved very difficult to organise. It's not easy to get together many different charities, all run by people with not enough funds and too much to do. VOCAL is now trying to get itself on a broader footing and to establish a constitution with elected committee members.

'It's gradually getting recognised and achieving publicity. It still has no permanent offices, but through recent funding from the DHSS it will be able to commission pamphlets and posters to promote the cause of the speech-handicapped. The present chairman is Mary La Fresnais, a full-time speech therapist in Kent.'

The conference drew together representatives from the Association for All Speech Impaired Children, the Association of Speech Clubs, the Association for Stammerers, British Dyslexia Association, Chest, Heart and Stroke Association, College of Speech Therapists, Invalid Children's Aid Association, National Autistic Society, National Association of Laryngectomee Clubs, National Society for Mentally Handicapped Children, Parkinson's Disease Society, Spastics Society and the WRVS; and also from such groups as the Study of Disorders in Human Communication and speech therapists in schools, relatives and parents, and specialists in associated branches of medicine.

Diana spoke for ten minutes. (She complained: *'Should be one hour for me – I speak so slowly!'*) As *the remedial therapist* summed up her speech: 'Miss Diana Law gave a rallying plea to those present, saying they must bully the DHSS into increasing facilities for communication with handicapped people.

'She spoke of demonstrations to save the whale, the publicity the stranded animals at Rome airport received, and then asked: *"But what about the speechless people?"* '

It marked just one more stage in her unceasing campaign.

19 From strength to strength

Diana's is a continuing story. The present marks only a stage in her determination to make an independent life for herself and claim the right to it for others.

With her 'miracle on a shoestring' she's already gone a long way. New speech clubs are continually being established here and overseas. The speech therapy programme is expanding. The Steering Group for the formation of an association for dysphasic adults is now, as she says, *'All set up and ready to go!'* In October 1979, inspired by the example of All Souls, thirteen other churches held their own service for the speech handicapped; and the moving prayer which closes this book was read in Sweden, Denmark, Norway, France, Belgium, Spain, Portugal, Germany, Australia, New Zealand, America, Canada, the Canary Islands, Jersey, Ireland and Northern Ireland, Greece and Malta. There is the possibility that, in the future, 'her' service may be televised.

She speaks on committees, visits clubs, addresses church groups. In 1980 she is to go to Sweden and Denmark to talk on speech clubs. Every time she makes more converts to her cause.

Gill Hodgson. 'Many years after her operation I heard her on the radio. That really made me prick up my ears! We always had too many patients to be able to keep in touch. Often we didn't know even whether they survived or not once they'd left. Diana didn't remember me at all, of course, but she said, "Lovely to meet you!" She came and visited me, and spoke at our church. It was a super evening. She handed out leaflets about her speech clubs.

'Her work is so important to people like herself. Doctors don't appreciate enough the problems dysphasics face. They have difficulties anyway in communicating with patients and relatives – and I'm not just thinking of the handicapped now. There's a parallel case where old people are concerned; Douglas Ritchie has touched on this in his "Problems of Aging" for the Open University. Old people have difficulties in communicating with doctors. It's a two-way process, with incomprehension on both sides. Relatives can be frightened and bewildered by details and by unknown factors. Doctors *think* their patients have understood what's been said, but they haven't. Fear shuts their ears.

'I believe something the same happens between speech-handicapped people, their relatives and doctors, with mis-understandings all round.'

Every time there appears an article which mentions her, or Alan Burgess's play receives another hearing abroad, letters flood in; Diana does her best to respond to them all. She feels a personal responsibility to each correspondent. To all of them – and many others – she sends an informative yearly newsletter.

Small gains are potentially enormous in effect. In January 1980, for the first time, Diana spoke at the Middlesex to medical students on the difficulties and feelings of the speech handicapped; for Diana, a breakthrough she had been seeking for many years. *'They listened well. It was a good day.'* In the future, she hopes to be speaking to them once a month.

On a more mundane level, her protests to the DHSS about her experiences at the Elephant and Castle produced results: a thorough new look at the facilities needed by the handicapped. Meanwhile, a letter promised, 'meetings attended by disabled people will be in Alexander Fleming House where car parking facilities and access are easier.' A small step in a never-ending struggle towards equality for the speech-handicapped.

In every way she can, Diana uses her life to help others. Each year she collects for Poppy Day, in the entrance of her block of flats, in others nearby, and in neighbouring shops. Twice (in 1979 and 1980) she organised and appeared on the BBC television programme *Lost for Words*. A television programme making use of her experiences is at present being planned for autumn, 1980. In mid-1979, with Joan Ellams and others at the CMRC, the Middlesex, and the Kingdom Ward Speech Therapy Trust, Diana helped the National Theatre with their production of Arthur Kopit's *Wings*, a play concerned with the problems of a speech-handicapped woman (Constance Cummings). Typically, Diana enjoyed meeting the cast, the preliminary work, the recording, but found the play itself too pessimistic. *'My message is hope,'* she said. *'Laughter, not tears. I want people to feel . . . a future.'*

And after her death, she hopes to continue to help. She has willed her body to the Middlesex Hospital and a sum of money for the use of the organs and research into the cause and effect of cerebral haemorrhage.

IN PERSONAL TERMS

Diana continues to improve in both speech and abilities. She has a great relish for life; loves parties and entertaining; goes out as much as she possibly can. She is immensely appreciative of the constant help and affection of all her friends, both male and female.

Lots of boy-friends then and still. Then, many men killed in action. In hospital, many come to see me. Not all. Some

*close friends now since stroke only see at parties. Illness
and tragedies they don't want to know.*

*Now lots more friends. But because of my mother, feel
I must be back by 11.30. Go out perhaps once a week.
Visiting. Parties.*

*Only one period since stroke. Never again sex. Before
that yes. Sex all gone. Very funny! Lots of kissing, but not
. . . very happy though.*

Diana fully appreciates that, financially, thanks to her
previous high earning capacity and her background, she has
been much better placed than most people recovering from
a stroke.

She had a series of well-paid jobs which allowed her to
save. When it became clear that she would never return to
her old job, ICL gave her a pension. She kept the same
pension for four years, and then received a rise. She also
receives a contribution from the state (still at present in a
state of flux).

But her expenses are heavy. She has kept on her own
flat to use as an occasional bolt-hole. Much of her income
goes to keep up with the mortgage payments, service charges
and rates on her mother's flat. Transport to visit essential
contacts like the Northcote Trust is also very expensive:
here her new mobility allowance, first paid in January 1980,
will help.

Her stroke affects her directly here as in other ways.
*'I like the Stock Exchange. I invest, I like shares, but not
any more. Can't read them.'* She was interested in the
financial side of business. Now she can no longer use that
experience.

But she knows that, compared with many, she is very
fortunate. *'Straitened circumstances, but very happy.'*

Her speech continues to improve.

Her language, defective though it is, is picturesque in
her use and choice of words. Her phrases convey the feel-

ing of someone who sees life in bold colours and attacks it with vigour.

'I'm going to write a stinker to him tonight.' 'You must chivy them.' 'I see the lie of the land.' 'I keep right on fighting.'

Michael Jackson. 'She's made tremendous progress, and I believe that she's still improving. I think that if she were tested at regular intervals, and if those tests were fine enough, you would detect a small but continual and steady improvement. Our former Principal used to test Douglas Ritchie in this way, and found that even years after his stroke he was continuing to progress.'

Joan Ellams. 'I would say that Diana has good communicating ability but very bad speech! She makes a limited vocabulary go a long way. She can sometimes express a whole complex sentence in a pepper-pot of words. She doesn't worry about sentence structure, or about grammar. Her use of tenses is unpredictable. She tends to speak in the present – then she leans one way to indicate the past, and the other way to mean the future. If she could resign herself to going more slowly, then she could pick her words more precisely. But her speech *works*.

'From her point of view none of this accuracy business worries her. *Efficiency* is Diana's watchword, and her speech is efficient. It's the same with her reading and writing. Her understanding of texts is good; tests show that she can read and understand quite complicated passages. She can't read aloud – that's a stumbling block. But she can read, quite adequately, as long as she takes it slowly. Mostly, she doesn't want to. She's impatient. She remembers how it used to be for her, and for her now it's not worth the time and effort it takes. I think if she thought it was, she would apply herself to it. Now she can get people to read her what matters. It's quicker, easier. More efficient.

'Its the same with writing. It's still very difficult for her. Her brief notes are cryptic – they rely on people getting them to understand – but they work. Anything more complicated means she has to look words up in her vocabulary and copy out letter by letter. It's a lot of effort and again takes a lot of time. It's not worth it, she thinks. She's got her scribes to help her, and it makes more sense to rely on them.'

Dr A-M T. 'What constantly astonishes me is how well she manages to communicate while she still has what is only, in fact, a very limited vocabulary. She compensates for it by her outgoingness. She's so open, so responsive, so smiling.

'She came not long ago to the preview of our new rehabilitation film. She stood up in the middle of the audience, without any preparation, and made a little speech. We were holding our breath, dreading that she might not manage it, but it came out perfectly. Quite spontaneously.

'Last year she came to help at our Bring and Buy. It was great watching her organise. She sent people here and there for markers and sellotape and so on, and told them what to charge. It's the same sort of organisation she brings to her cause.'

Betty Giles. 'She's made great progress over the five years I've known her. She couldn't write at all then, or converse on the telephone. Now she holds conversations easily. She never fails to surprise me. She says she can't think, her brain won't work, but it works quicker than mine! If something's happened during the week, when I get there she's all ready to pick it up. She's always got her eye open for anyone who will help her cause.'

Moira Tighe. 'Diana has enormous charm. She never talks about her illness, though she must often be in a lot of pain. She loves entertaining; her scribes get liberally dosed with sherry! She knows what she wants, and she knows how to get what she wants. She has enormous self-confidence. She almost blackmails people into doing things. She gets them almost eating out of her hand. In the end they say yes, because it's easier than saying no.'

'NEVER MIND! ALWAYS SOMETHING!'

Diana's oldest friends and family, who can look back and compare the different stages of her life, all emphasise the same elements.

Jacqueline Morrell. 'Diana's letter to the *Telegraph* really sparked her off. It gave direction to her life. She has enormous character. Great courage. It would be so easy to become shut in oneself, but Diana hasn't. She remains open to others. She's remarkable. She gets so much fun and pleasure out of life.

'Today of course she's almost completely independent. All I do for her are her toe-nails and finger-nails and some of her shopping. A lot of her friends – most of her friends – have been wonderful. There've been others who've dropped off, so she only hears from them at Christmas and times like that. But then I suppose that happens anyway as life goes on. And she's made many more since she was ill.

'Looking back, I'd say I feel now that I neglected my husband and my daughter. But how can you say that? It's not easy. Whatever you do, you fail somewhere. It wasn't easy for us, it wasn't easy for Diana either. The awful frustration that she felt often burst out of her. You can imagine it – being trapped inside and not being able to get across what you feel. There were terrible scenes over being five minutes late, demanding things, orders. For an intelligent, vital person like Diana, it must have been intolerable.

'I was lucky in many ways. After Coventry, all during the worst days, I had six years in *No Sex Please We're British*. It was a super job. Without that as an anchor. . . .

'I know Diana always thinks of the relatives. Maybe her book will explain things a bit to them.'

G

Faith Porter. 'I can't think of a friend it could have crippled more. She has a very strong faith now, but I don't think really that she had then. She had nothing peaceful to support her. No quiet interests at all. But she has something of the same courage and determination and sheer *obstinacy* of Douglas Bader.'

Anne Handley-Derry. 'Simply by existing she gives heart to people. Not just those recovering from strokes, but others who aren't physically afflicted in any way, but can respond to her courage and determination.

'It's impossible to imagine the frustration Diana must face every day. To be virtually unable to read and write. To know exactly what you want to say, but not be able to get it across. Her language is not precise enough, though her thoughts are. What we gather is often only an approximation.

'But she has immense guts. She's just put her mind to it, and plodded on. She's shown tremendous patience. When I first knew her, she had a really sharp, almost acid sense of humour. She was impatient, never tolerated fools gladly. She's a much finer person now than ever she was. I'm astonished at the strength and patience she's shown. She's been through so much, yet she's hardly ever broken down.

'A lot has changed in the last few years since Diana had her stroke. I think people generally are far more aware of strokes and what happens to people who are trying to recover. Even so, there's a long way to go.

'My son has recently qualified as a doctor, and he tells me that in all his medical training the importance of speech therapy and what it can achieve was hardly touched on. As for ordinary people in the street, especially if they don't themselves know anyone who's had a stroke, they don't know how to respond to someone who has difficulty in speaking.

'What we need is a way to indicate to others that there

is a disability – the equivalent of a white stick for blind people. Perhaps a bracelet of some sort. The trouble is that there's rather a lot to get over: "I'm not an idiot, I can understand, I can respond, but please let me take my time." And of course people's capacities vary. We need to go on educating the public into understanding what's involved.

'That's why Diana has to be single-minded. Her cause is an obsession. She'll never be satisfied as long as there's anyone anywhere needing speech therapy and not getting it.

'She always stresses the role of the supportive family. She knows how much the stroke patient has to rely on the help of relatives, and how much toll this takes of them, but she's not always ready to recognise that they have needs too, to make allowances for the other demands on them. It's not easy to achieve a sort of balance.

'So when she gets to be her most over-bearing – and she knows what I think, because I've told her so, she usually takes it from me after all these years – it's not significant compared to her achievements.

'Especially when I think that whenever there's a set-back, Diana shrugs her shoulders, laughs, and says, "Never mind! Always something!" '

'A MARTYR TO THE CAUSE'

Yvonne Edels is particularly well qualified by her un-usual relationship with Diana over the past years to give an interesting perspective not only on Diana herself but on the problems too of other dysphasics.

Yvonne Edels qualified as a speech therapist in 1971 after a three-year course at Birmingham Speech Therapy Training School (now part of the Birmingham Polytechnic), which had been open for only one year. She was one of seven 'on a guinea-pig course, an advantage in many ways.' After qualifying she worked for six months in Cardiff, then came south to work part-time in the Middlesex Hospital and part-time in an

ILEA post in Tooting concerned with very handicapped children. In 1976 she started working full-time at the Middlesex as Head of the Speech Therapy Department.

'I've never treated Diana, but I've had a lot of contact with her since first meeting her seven years ago. We have an unusual relationship: she's not quite a patient, not quite a professional, but something between the two. I've used her to demonstrate in lectures, helped check reports of interviews for her and been on radio programmes with her, and I sit with her on committees, including VOCAL.

'She's a unique person because of a combination of circumstances: her own personality, her professional background, her family, her religious faith, her wide acquaintance with people in politics and industry. She's a remarkable person who's done remarkable things. She used to have political ambitions, and I know she stood as candidate in both local and national elections. But since her stroke she's done more for more people than she would ever have achieved as a councillor or MP.

'She deals with enormous problems in discomfort and often in pain. She suffers great frustration, and has learnt to come to terms with it. She has immense energy. It takes many stroke patients, even with the help of a spouse, virtually all their time to get up, get dressed, get fed, and simply handle the basics of living. Diana does all this and all her own work too: her letters, her committees, her phone calls and so on.

'In the course of her crusade, Diana has done more for the cause of the adult dysphasic than any other single person, including top speech therapists. She can open doors others people can't. Because of her speech handicap and her own experiences, she gets listened to where other people might not be. She is totally dedicated to her cause, and totally single-minded. In her business life before her stroke, she must have been used to being kicked in the teeth and bouncing back again. She uses the same grit and determination now.

'At the same time, this cause is what keeps her going. It gives her something to do, she goes ahead and does it, and she gets a come-back from it. We all need it. I think in the caring profession we all love to be loved, especially in our early days. We need the feed-back to keep us going. It's the same with Diana.

'The same persistence which brings results can however also present problems. Plans for actions are all controlled by speech. We rely on the subtle choice of words to convey the finesse of a situation. For dysphasics, this may not always be possible. Because they have difficulty in word-finding and sentence construction, they may be unable to be as diplomatic as they would wish. This can create major difficulties for their relatives, who may feel, for example, that they are on the receiving end of orders rather than requests.

'This aspect may present obstacles for Diana. The further she progresses, and the more demands are made on her, the more she needs to exercise moderation and diplomacy.

'Diana also demonstrates another predicament faced by those who have had strokes, which is a decreased capacity to control emotion. She has come to handle her feelings much better, but if a number of things combine to go wrong she can still react with tears – as she wouldn't have done previously. This is a direct result of the stroke and the damage caused to the brain. I can feel something of the same thing myself at the moment. I'm pregnant, and I know that I now over-react. My tolerance is displaced. I don't feel things any differently, but I feel them more strongly; I express them in ways I wouldn't normally, and I feel my sense of perspective has shifted.

'It's something like that for people who have suffered a stroke. It can be very difficult to explain to relatives. Sometimes they come to me and say there's been a personality change. *No.* It isn't that. It's the way in which that personality is *expressed* which has changed. Relatives can find this very distressing. It's especially difficult when it's men who are affected. In our culture, people don't get so upset at women bursting into tears, but they do when it's a husband or father who might before never have cried in years. They have to accept that this is part of the stroke.'

'Diana is a great organiser. She's very good at getting people to do what she wants them to do. At her behest I found myself spending a week of my holiday writing an article for the Editor of GLAD (Greater London Association for the Disabled). Part of me resented giving up my free time in this way, but I'm glad I did it, and I would never have done it without her insistence. On the other hand, she sometimes wants things done which are effectively not possible, and she can find it hard to accept this. She urges me to run a speech group at the Middlesex. I would willingly do it if possible, but there simply aren't enough dysphasics within reach. This is a Central London teaching hospital, with only a small living-in population. We get patients from all over. Dysphasics are frequently physically handicapped as well, and transport is a problem. I do have a laryngectomy group, because there is a large number of them and they're mobile. But I have only a very small core of available dysphasic patients. I have tried to run a group, but it didn't work; there were only three people turning up.

'But as far as the actual problem of dysphasia is concerned, I can only echo Diana's song. There is too little time and money spent on dysphasia; all the concentration goes on the physical side. Once a patient is continent and can move around, he or she can go home – no matter what their state of mind or whether they can speak or not. This is true even of someone living on their own.

'One of our difficulties, as a profession, is that the effectiveness of speech therapy is judged by its results, but that until we have the opportunity to practise it as extensively as it demands the results will not be forthcoming. Compared with the support given to physiotherapy and occupational therapy, that given to speech therapy is negligable. We at the Middlesex are not badly off, but even so we have only two full-time speech therapists to cope with the demand from a proportion of patients occupying 700 beds. If we had a speech therapist on each ward, speech therapy could get in there first and start right away.

'Nobody shouts at physiotherapists if they can't get arms and legs working immediately. They understand that it will take time, that patients have to be taught to compensate for damaged muscles and nerves. But people – both ordinary people and in the medical profession – don't see brain damage in the same way. Yet the repair work, the compensatory work, is far more complex.

'Language is the highest intellectual function that we know. In spite of this, speech therapists are expected to rehabilitate a damaged system in forty-five minutes once or twice a week.

'A further complication is that speech therapy is not passive. Physiotherapy can be. There are ways in which you can exercise a patient's muscles without direct co-operation. But speech therapy, to succeed, must have the patient's co-operation; and it invariably demands a high degree of concentration. Those recovering from strokes lack this. They tire easily. If a patient doesn't get to see a speech therapist until after 3 pm it's time wasted. There's no chance of getting through to them. The energy is gone.

'Many doctors still feel that speech recovery is spontaneous, and that speech therapists are just playing games. We know this isn't so, but we need the chance to prove it. We need an enormous educational programme, not only for the public, but for the medical profession too.

'Diana is trying to do this, using herself as a model. She's getting across to nursing people, speech therapists, and laymen; but I feel that she's not yet – with rare exceptions

– communicating with consultants: Dr S at the CMRC is unique in his understanding of these problems.

'Here at the Middlesex we are starting to improve the educational side. We're now lecturing to nurses, with Diana's help, to medical students – as part of the geriatric course – to physiotherapists and physiotherapy students and to outside people. We need much more. At present speech therapy is *not* adequate. When you've had your stroke, and it's happened to you, you can't do anything about it. There's never enough money: we're failing to get across that what's spent on speech therapy is cost-effective. Rehabilitation *saves* money in the long run.

'Possibly the greatest wish of dysphasics is to be accepted by others as the same ordinary individuals they were before their stroke. Too often those they meet draw away in embarrassment. They may be considered drunk, stupid or mad. We need a campaign to educate the public to be as sensitive to the needs of the speech-handicapped as they are to those of the blind or deaf.

'As I recently wrote: *"It seems ironic that those people who suffer most are the very ones who, by virtue of their disability, are the least able to agitate for more to be done."*

'That's why someone like Diana is so important.

'There are two things to be said simultaneously. The first is that she has done more for adult dysphasics than anyone else. The second is that, without her stroke, she would have gone much further much sooner. There's a personal loss on the one hand, and on the other immense gain for the many people she's succeeded in helping, both directly and indirectly.

'She's a tremendous catalyst. Her criteria are dynamic and dogmatic. She decides what she wants, how to get it, who to approach, where to get the money. The people she approaches can't just brush her off. Because of her speech defect, they have to listen to her, and once they've listened, most often they act.

'Her faith keeps her going. It's a powerful element in her life.

'Diana is a martyr to the cause. Hats off to her! What she's done is unparalelled. She has all my admiration.'

Diana and her mother both see her life since her stroke as gain, not loss; each appreciates the qualities in the other's character which have made this possible.

Without my mother . . . nothing. She is very tired now, but very brave. And lots of young people and conversation . . . My stroke changed me. I cry a very lot of the time. Tears are the effect of the stroke. In hospital I cried four times a day. At the Wolfson once a day. At Camden twice a week. Now – once a month! Sometimes I cross. But now I cross at way of handicapped, not cross about anything else. Life . . . good.

As Diana once said to Daphne Stafford, she wouldn't have had her life any different. Daphne Stafford herself comments: 'She is creating of it a positive achievement.'

Mary Law. 'It's true that if I hadn't been here, or if I hadn't been the sort of person I am, Diana's life might have been very different. But I've never been one for hysterics. I'm proud of the fact that three of my five children have won awards for bravery. All my life I have just had to follow what was in front of me.

'I couldn't have lived with her before her stroke, but afterwards it was all right. Before she had a different temperament. Very vivacious, plenty of men-friends, successful, fault-finding sometimes. Afterwards, she didn't find fault, less vivacious perhaps, but incredibly patient. And always happy. God sent her the compensation of helping others.

'I had to give up my painting, my voluntary activities . . . I have sometimes felt imprisoned. But I never thought of not doing what I had to do. I know some people thought I was unfeeling because I didn't go round weeping and wailing. Real grief is quiet.

'When tragedy hits you, either you lie down.

'Or you stand up.

'That's all there is to it.'

Epilogue

Appendix I

A SELECTION OF RELEVANT BOOKS: some are out of print, but are usually obtainable through libraries.

Stroke, by Douglas Ritchie: Faber & Faber, 1974. A personal account, in his own words, by a stroke victim at the CMRC. (See above p. 78).

A Stroke in the Family, by Valerie Eaton Griffith: Wildwood House, London, 1975. An account (with lessons and exercises) by a neighbour-turned-teacher of how actress Patricia Neal and writer Alan Moorehead were helped to speak again after a stroke. (See above p. 174).

Learning to Speak After a Stroke, by Charles R. Isted: King Edward's Hospital Fund for London, 1979. A large-type book on a spiral binding by a speech-handicapped stroke patient; advice from his own experiences for patients and relatives, with exercises and aids for speech and understanding.

Speak for Yourself, by Betty Brown: Educational Explorers, Reading, 1971. A personal view of speech therapy as a career, with details of what can be done for the speech-handicapped both here and in the States.

The Third Killer, by Guy Wint: Chatto & Windus, 1965. A stroke is the third most common cause of death: an autobiographical view by a journalist.

Help Yourselves, by Peggy Jay: Ian Henry Publications, 1979. A spiral-hinged handbook with a great deal of practical information for hemiplegics and their families; brief sections on speech and writing.

Appendix II

SOME ASSOCIATIONS CONCERNED WITH THE SPEECH-HANDICAPPED

College of Speech Therapists: 2/47 St John's Wood High Street, London NW8.

Chest, Heart and Stroke Association: Tavistock House North, Tavistock Square, London WC1.

National Association of Laryngectomee Clubs: Fourth Floor, Michael Sobell House, 30 Dorset Square, London NW1 6QL.

Parkinson's Disease Society: 81 Queens Road, London SW19 8NR.

Association for All Speech Impaired Children (AFASIC): 347 Central Markets, Smithfield, London EC1A 9NH.

Steering Group for an association for dysphasic adults: Cicely Northcote Trust, Northcote House, Royal Street, London SE1. (See p. 182).

Association of Stammerers: 86 Blackfriars Road, London SE1.

A Directory of Stroke Clubs is available from the Chest, Heart and Stroke Association, but only some of these will have the help of speech therapists.

A Register of Speech Clubs is available from the Cicely Northcote Trust. (See above).

Please contact the above for current details.

Appendix III

Information on speech therapy as a career is obtainable from the College of Speech Therapists, the Department of Health and Social Security, Area Health Authorities, or any of the following training establishments.

TRAINING ESTABLISHMENTS
DIPLOMA COURSES

CITY OF BIRMINGHAM POLYTECHNIC

School of Speech Therapy, Department of Science, Franchise Street, Perry Barr, Birmingham B42 2US. Tel: 021 356 6911. Head of School: Miss J. Stengelhofen, LCST, DTST.

THE CENTRAL SCHOOL OF SPEECH AND DRAMA

Embassy Theatre, 64 Eton Avenue, Swiss Cottage, London NW3 3HY. Tel: 01 722 8183. Director of Speech Therapy: Mrs Elaine Hodkinson, LCST.

LEICESTER POLYTECHNIC

School of Speech Pathology, Scraptoft Campus, Scraptoft, Leicester LE7 9SU. Tel: 0533 431011: office ext. 279. Head of School: Miss E. G. Barlow, MSc, LCST: ext. 281.

SCHOOL FOR THE STUDY OF DISORDERS OF HUMAN COMMUNICATION

86 Blackfriars Road, London SE1. Tel: 01 928 4563. Senior Lecturer: Mrs Margaret Fawcus, MSc, LCST.

DEGREE COURSES ARE AVAILABLE AS FOLLOWS (APPLICATION THROUGH U.C.C.A.)

BSc Hons (Speech)

The University of Newcastle-upon-Tyne, Speech Unit, Further Professional Studies Division, School of Education, St Thomas' Street, Newcastle-upon-Tyne NE1 7RU. Tel: Newcastle 28511 ext. 3451. Head of School: Professor Dennis Child, BSc, MEd, PhD, FBPsS. Enquiries to Course Co-ordinator: Dr R. Lesser, BA, BSc, PhD.

BEd, BEd Hons (Speech Pathology and Therapeutics)

Jordanhill College of Education, School of Speech Therapy, 76 Southbrae Drive, Glasgow G13 1PP. Tel: 041 959 1232. Director: Miss A. R. Wallace, MSc (Purdue), LCST.

BSc Hons (Speech Pathology and Therapy)

University of Manchester, Department of Audiology and Education of the Deaf, Manchester M13 9PL. Tel: 061 272 3333 ext. 3152. Tutor to the Course: Mrs B. Byers Brown, MEd, MCST.

BA Linguistics and Language Pathology (Speech Therapy)

Department of Linguistic Science, University of Reading, Whiteknights, Reading, Berkshire. Course Director: Professor D. Crystal, BA, PhD.

BSc (Speech Therapy) (CNAA degree)

Speech Therapy Division, Ulster Polytechnic, Jordanstown, Newtownabbey, Co Antrim BT37 0QB. Tel: 0231 65131. Senior Course Tutor: Miss Mary Thomas, LCST, DTST: ext. 2140.

BSc (Speech Therapy) (CNAA degree)

Leeds Polytechnic. School of Health and Applied Sciences, Speech Therapy Section, Calverley Street, Leeds LS1 3HE. Tel: 0532 46240/941. Course Director: Miss F. M. Jones, MSc, LCST. Head of School: Dr K. R. Fell, BPharm, PhD, FPS, MIBiol.

BSc Speech Pathology and Therapy

City of Manchester College of Higher Education, School of Speech Therapy, Hathersage Road, Manchester M13 0JA. Tel: 061 225 9054. Principal Lecturer in Speech Pathology: Mrs J. S. Lambert, MSc, BSc (Speech).

BMed Sci (Speech)

The University, Sheffield S10 2TN. Further information and enquiries to: Miss D. A. Treharne, MSc, LCST, Department of Linguistics, The University, Sheffield S10 2NT. Tel: 0742 785555 ext. 702.

BA (Remedial Linguistics)

School of Remedial Linguistics, University of Dublin, Trinity College, Dublin 2. Tel: 772941. Head of School: Sister Marie de Montfort Supple, MPhil, DTST, LCST. Deputy: Mrs D. Walker, MSc, LCST, ALAM.

BSc in Speech Pathology and Therapy

Queen Margaret College, School of Speech Therapy, Clerwood Terrace, Edinburgh EH12 8TS. Tel: 031 3398111. Head of School: Miss A. M. McGovern, MA, LCST.

BSc Hons (Speech Sciences)

University College, London, Gower Street, London WC1E 6BT in collaboration with The National Hospitals College of Speech Sciences, 59 Portland Place, London W1N 3AJ. Principal: Dr Jean M. Cooper, PhD, LCST.

BSc Hons in Speech Therapy

Cardiff School of Speech Therapy, South Glamorgan Institute of Higher Education, Llandaff Centre, Western Avenue, Cardiff CF5 2YB. Tel: 0222 567345. Director of Studies: Carol J. Miller, MSc, LCST.